Cícera Paz
Ítalo Marcos

The Siting Trash Syndrome in Systems and Genetics

Cícera Paz
Ítalo Marcos

The Siting Trash Syndrome in Systems and Genetics

Rubbish and Genetics

ScienciaScripts

Imprint
Any brand names and product names mentioned in this book are subject to trademark, brand or patent protection and are trademarks or registered trademarks of their respective holders. The use of brand names, product names, common names, trade names, product descriptions etc. even without a particular marking in this work is in no way to be construed to mean that such names may be regarded as unrestricted in respect of trademark and brand protection legislation and could thus be used by anyone.

Cover image: www.ingimage.com

This book is a translation from the original published under ISBN 978-620-2-03126-4.

Publisher:
Sciencia Scripts
is a trademark of
Dodo Books Indian Ocean Ltd. and OmniScriptum S.R.L publishing group

120 High Road, East Finchley, London, N2 9ED, United Kingdom
Str. Armeneasca 28/1, office 1, Chisinau MD-2012, Republic of Moldova, Europe
Printed at: see last page
ISBN: 978-620-8-35255-4

SUMMARY

INTRODUCTION

Mitotic Waste and Mater Contractile Cells are two concepts that are totally unknown in **current medical literature**. This book provides a very clear definition of both concepts, as well as a lot of information about concepts that physiology has been talking about since the beginning, and which have now been given a new connotation, a new meaning and a new guise. Antigens are in no way harmful to our body, DNA is just DN because it doesn't contain acids, base nuclei and a reverse strand in our organism, the Sensory Energy System led by Purkinje, and led by Granule Cells, new systems are known and others unified, the formation of Alpha Delta, and the child, with super powers, these and many other pieces of information will be given to the reader in this book.

Genetics and other systems get a new look with this book and the reader will learn who the Mater Contractile Cells are, and why only five pairs of cells are responsible for all the commands in the organism. Who these cells are and what they do, the reader will now know, and what's more, why science has never talked about the energetic command system in our body? In the unfolding and coding of these cells, the reader will learn why some systems have merged in this work. Genetics and the immune system are the key and the lock to understanding or explaining countless diseases in any part of the body. The LS is responsible for an infinite number of pathologies, and this book answers many questions raised in current medical literature, from cancer, diabetes, mental illnesses, deformities in genetics, rheumatic diseases and other pathologies lodged in the human organism.

Lixo Sitiante is therefore a cosmic dust that appears in the form of a mass in the body, like cement dust on a leaf, and so it appears in the cell acting as a very potent poison affecting the structure of the cellular system whether in the membrane, the synovial fluid, the ligaments, or even inside the cell in its various segments. It enters man through the sacral foramen up to the L5 level, becoming invasive at this point, into the spinal cord where it accompanies the cerebrospinal fluid that runs longitudinally through it, bridging the brainstem, and can be clearly seen in the pyramidal decursion arriving at the median opening of the IV ventricle, it crosses between the III ventricle and the lateral ventricles, reaching the arachnoid granulapses via the superior sargital sinus and thus falling into the bloodstream, acting in a chain from there on ten systems in our organism, namely:

Functional Breakdown of Organizational Systems

Central Energetic Circulatory Sensory System (AaBb-Dd-Ff-Hh-Jj) Central Sensory System for Commanding MCCs (AaBb-Dd-Ff-Hh-Jj) Unified Nervous and Muscular System (Aa-Bb-Cc-Dd-Ee-Ff)
Circulatory System (Blood, Lymphatic, Hormonal, Respiratory) (Aa- Bb-c-d-e-f-g-h-i-j)
Unified Articular Skeletal System (Aa-Bb-Cc-Dd-Ee-Ff-)
Unified Immune System and Genetics (Aa-Bb-Dd-Ff-Hh-Jj-Mm-Oo-Qq)
Integumentary system (touch, pressure, hearing, sight, taste, vibration, cold, heat, pain)(Aa-Bb-c-d-f-h-j-m-o-)

Note: The breakdown of these systems can be found in the fifth chapter of this book, **Principles of the Nervous System.**

In Genetics, LS modifies the cell's DNA, causing mutations, errors in the various stages of transcription and translation, causing structural changes in the genomic DNA, thus giving rise to chromosomal abnormalities such as: Trisomy of the autosomes such as: Trisomy 21 (Down's Syndrome); Trisomy 18 Syndrome, Trisomy 13 Syndrome where the authors of this event say that the underlying cause of the non-disjunction in the event is unclear, claiming that Down's is more common in the offspring of older mothers. In reality, at an older age there is in fact a greater accumulation of LS in the body, which the reader will understand better as he gets to know this work.

In the brain, LS, which is responsible for removing sodium from the body, causes various types of damage such as: Alzhaimer's disease, dementia, Parkson's disease, multiple sclerosis, forgetfulness, slow thinking, and the person who has a large accumulation of LS is as if they were in slow motion, working as if they were working at only 40% of their potential. LS is fully visible in apoptosis, and enzymes are a kind of receptor and carrier magnet in the body, an example being caspases.

In the respiratory system, the effects of LS on chronic obstructive pulmonary disease (COPD) are a warning of the dangers posed by the action of this waste on the functioning of the organism as a whole, especially in the lungs. It has been responsible for a very high percentage of illnesses found in physiology and neurology textbooks, where the authors generally fail to find an explanation for certain illnesses, such as multiple sclerosis, alzhaimer, parkkson, eplepsy, etc.

Maternal Contractile Cells Who are they?

Our whole body works in **antithesis**, in a **closed circle,** but the ones responsible for this intense work are five pairs of cells (**Maternal Contractile Cells**) that are part of a larger group of command cells; twelve pairs of cells that are still unknown to current science in the way they act in the organism. The MCCs, then, are a tiny population of five pairs of cells that always work in pairs and as a team, in an orderly and alternating fashion, maternal grandparents, paternal grandparents, in ribbons that unfold in all the systems in a quantity specific to each system. They are extremely precise and cohesive in all their work. They work in ten systems in our body, they are cells that are harmful to the body. This tiny population always works as a team and in pairs, acting in different ways in each system.

It is an organized, rational, precise, coherent and highly specialized team that is responsible for all action, contraction, nerve synapses, reflex movements, blood circulation, closed circuits and open chains, motor coordination, gas exchange, respiration, afferent and efferent, in short, wherever there is action, there are the **contractile Mater Cells** present throughout our body and which appear in all the functioning of the vital systems.

They have an extraordinary ability to optically read everything and everyone that surrounds us up to the tenth generation and are responsible for the entire command of vital functions in our organism.

There are six pairs of cells, the first of which **(Aa), (Alpha)** is formed by the father and mother and in some systems appears together with **Beta (Bb**) forming a single cellular unit. In some systems such as the circulatory system, the immune system and in genetics etc. we will find **Alpha and Beta** together in a single unit, they are the parents and maternal grandparents. You can observe the distribution of these cells in the dendrites in neurons, or in the pyramids in the kidneys or in other vital organs.

In Genetics, they are treated by chromosomes and only in this system and in the immune system will we find 24 units of **Mater Contractile Cells** (MCCs), which are confused by the authors as being **23 pairs of chromosomes**, and which in reality, the pair of Alpha chromosomes are two in one, and are often even four in one as in the heart, where Alpha and Beta are together, that is father and mother and maternal grandparents.

The MCCs have specific names given by the authors in each system, but the reader will understand that these cells are exactly the same in some systems, and all of this will be explained in detail so that the reader has no doubts. They feature prominently in Genetics, for their typically maternal role, and in the Immune System, which is a system in which these cells work beautifully, communicating and observing each other to know who is entering and leaving our bodies. They work like radar systems, and what is most incredible is their high capacity for memorization, as is the case with **antigens** in our favor and which are mistaken by researchers as intruders in our organism.

The immune system fights an intense battle to expel the invader.

This study will only present these cellular units in five systems, namely: Cardiac System, Immune System, and in genetics, respiratory and integumentary, in reality the organism has only seven systems; the other organs, or cells are accessory, the reader will also learn more about this subject.

The role of the CCMS is to be found in all systems, and it will be necessary for the reader to know how they are broken down and functionally mapped in order to better understand this study.

Informative mapping of the sculptural and functional pattern of ten cell units in our organism (Mater Contractile Cells) or MCCs.

Cell		
Aa Alfha (father and mother) are always together		(Aa) Alfha
B cell (the maternal grandparent)	**B** cell (maternal grandmother)	(Bb) Beta
C cell (paternal grandfather)	Cell **c** (paternal grandmother)	(Cc) Ceci
D cell (maternal grandparent)	**D** cell (maternal grandparent)	(Dd) DELTA
Cell E (paternal grandfather)	Cell **e** (paternal grandmother)	(Ee) E Reverse
F cell (maternal grandparent)	**F** cell (maternal grandparent)	(Ff) Hexa Mater
G cell (paternal grandfather)	Cell g (paternal grandmother)	(Gg) Mater G
H cell (maternal grandparent)	Cell h (maternal grandparent)	(Hh) Mater holy
Cell I (paternal grandfather)	Celula Ii (paternal grandmother)	(Ii) Mater I
J cell (maternal grandparent)	Jj cell (maternal grandmother)	(Jj) jota holy
Celula L (paternal grandfather)	Cell Ll (paternal grandmother)	(Ll) Mater L
M cell (maternal grandparent)	Mm cell (maternal grandparent)	(Mm) Mater M
Cell N (Paternal Grandfather)	Nn cell (paternal grandmother)	(Nn) Mater N
O-Cell (Maternal Grandparent)	Mm cell (maternal grandparent)	(Mm) Mater M
Pp cell (paternal grandfather)	Pp cell (paternal grandmother)	(Pp) Mater P
Qq cell (maternal grandparent)	Qq cell (maternal grandmother)	(Qq) Mater Q

Cell Rr (paternal grandfather)	Rr cell (paternal grandmother)	Mater R
Ss cell (maternal grandparent)	Ss cell (maternal grandparent)	Mater Ss

Attention - the number of MSCs is 23 pairs, which are the chromosomes in Genetics, the control cells are five pairs, but only of deoxyribose cells, the other two pairs are good cells for the organism, but after the letter ESSE they are already harmful cells, which will form macrophages, Glia cells etc. in the organism. It is for this reason that embryos passing through these cells in their formation (cell number 21 or chromosome pair 21) run the risk of being born with deficiencies and deformities, as in Down's Syndrome. The number of cells will depend on certain systems and their functionality. The important thing to know is that these are five pairs of good cells (**AaBb-Dd-Ff-Hh-Jj), which** are deoxyribose cells that function throughout the body. In genetics and the immune system, they work in a total of 23 pairs of maternal contractile cells, and the reader will have all the information he needs on the breakdown of these cells a little further on. All the information in these cells is passed on through the **conductivity** process in the purkinje fibers in cells Aa, Bb, Cc, Dd, Ee, Ff, Gg, Hh, Ii, Jj. All the electrical properties work around the commands of these cells. Each pair of these cells is driven by specific gases; we have the set of maternal grandparents, the set of maternal grandparents, the set of maternal grandparents, the set of paternal grandparents, and whether they act together or separately, these groups therefore carry specific gases, oxygen, nitrogen, hydrogen, so oxygen the parents and all the grandparents and nitrogen, the parents and all the grandparents.

CHAPTER I

MAPPING INFORMATION ON THE SHAPE AND SCULPTURE OF MATER CONTRACTILE CELLS IN THE CIRCULATORY SYSTEM

In the heart, these highly specialized contractile cells receive commands from up to 10 genes always in pairs, i.e. from Aa to Jj . They pass this information on to the pairs Aa, Bb, Cc, Dd, Ee and Ff, Gg, Hh, Ii, Jj through the process of conductivity and purkinje fibers that can issue any type of command; either from the inside out, efferences, or from the outside in, afferences, and a kind of remote control, where one person can send any type of command to another and receive it at the same time. In this way, it is possible for any individual to know the cellular command of the other up to the tenth generation. But attention, this is only possible in this system; knowing that the command of these cells are in ten systems in our organism. The **circulatory system**, together with **genetics,** are like a **key and a lock** in our organism. Genetics would be the gateway to all the other systems. In this way, we can say that one processes and the other emits control over the other systems through afferent and efferent commands.

The arteries are constant targets of destructive commands coming from the afferent pathways, and in recent times these commands have multiplied, along with diseases linked to the heart. Therefore, heart-related diseases or pulmonary disorders are actually commands sent via the **contractile mater cells** in the heart.

The heart is made up of cubes in which all the Mater cells are involved. In the first cube there are the Alfha Aa cells (formed by the father and mother) and the Be Bb cells (maternal grandparents) and also the Cc Ceci cells (paternal grandparents), which according to the authors are the **cardiac pacemakers** and are so called because they generate a lot of force; In the second atrial cube we have Dd Delta (second generation maternal grandparents or Bizavos) and in the third atrial cube we have Ee E Reversa Hexa Mater (maternal and paternal grandparents), this force is located in the cube that the authors call "NO AV" but in reality it is an atrial cube. Thus, this hub complements the previous forge and continues the cardiac cycle through the conduction process of these cells.

In this study, this Dd (Delta) cell pair is very important, as it is an indicator of a child's genius, i.e. if the fetus was given two maternal grandparents, the child will be born a genius, as it has eight brains coupled into one. The reader will understand this a little further on.

The most important work in the body is carried out by the **Ff (Hexa Mater)** cells. They are considered the common base, or **base Q/B** group, which means "**I want to** be **well"** because these cells are always working attentively on behalf of the body so that the individual can always be well and healthy, but they have to contend with another group of Reverse cells, which, as their name suggests, are always doing the opposite work, except for the **Reverse "Ee"**, which can be for or against the body.

It is a reverse cell, but still belongs to the basic Q/B group. There is a remnant of Mater cells that are released into the **Genetic System**, and will appear in the **Immune System** and be sent to other organs when necessary. These remaining Mater cells can work in antagonism to the organism itself, and this will be observed there in the immune system and in Genetics. This study brings new concepts in Physiology, unknown until now by current science, here is a new study in Human Physiology, with more clarification and more understanding for many diseases, and behaviors in the organ system.

The last cells of the common base or Q/B base are in charge of the lower, heavier services, they are the pairs of cells **(Ee) E Reversas** paternal grandparents, and **(Ff) Hexa Mater** which are the maternal grandparents.

Attention - Mater cells from Aa (Alfha) to Jj (J Mater,) are not harmful to the organism if they are on the maternal ribbon, i.e. (Aa-Bb-Dd-Ff-Hh-Jj), but paternal Mater cells can be reversed from Ee, i.e. (Aa-Cc-Ee-Gg- Ii) are acidic and can cause damage or not to the organism depending exclusively on the ribbon that makes them up in the formation of the Mater Contractile Cells. They always appear alternately and always end in maternal grandparents, these are the last pairs of terminal cells of these cellular units and these last two sets of cells in the organism work differently, and their functions will be explained in detail as being inferior and separate from the others.

These cells act differently in terms of their number in genetics, and this will be explained in the chapter on genetics. In the heart, they are differentiated when they join Aa Bb, Cc in a single block, so they organize themselves in the way they need to function.

> *"The heart illustrated on page 9-1 is actually made up of two separate pumps: the right heart, which pumps blood to the lungs, and the left heart, which pumps blood to the peripheral organs. In turn, each of these hearts is a two-chamber pulsatile pump made up of an atrium and a ventricle. Each atrium is a weak primer pump for the ventricle, helping to propel the blood into it. The ventricles in turn provide the main pumping force that propels the blood through the pulmonary circulation from the right ventricle or the peripheral circulation from the left ventricle." Guyton and Hall pg. 107*

Muscle contraction in the heart lasts longer than any skeletal muscle because its functionality is different from other muscles, which only need to contract.

The heart isn't two pumps, as Guyton informs us, it's a muscle, the most important of them all because its work is exceptionally different from the others in our skeleton, and it has an autonomous form of contraction. These hubs work with great force, and the first atrial hub is called the Cardiac Pacemaker by the authors, because the parents and maternal grandparents work together there to process more force.

> *"In addition, cardiac muscle contains myofibrils with actin and myosin filaments almost identical to those found in skeletal muscle" Guyton pg 107.*

Attention, actin and myosin belong to the same group of cells that was discussed at the beginning of this work; actin belongs to the Q/B deoxyribose group, they are the parents and maternal grandparents and myosin is the paternal grandparent. This group of cells (Mater Contractile Cells) will appear throughout the Physiology literature under different names, but they are always command cells. An example to clarify things for the reader is Cytosine, which is all the maternal grandparents, Guanine, which is all the maternal grandparents, Thymine, which is all the paternal grandparents, Adenine, which is all the maternal grandparents, So, depending on where these cells are, this study will identify for the reader who they are, who the Maternal Contractile Cells are, which in reality are just four groups, namely maternal grandparents, paternal grandparents, maternal grandparents, paternal grandparents, plus the father, mother and maternal grandparents.

The author also talks about the opening of the sodium and potassium channels, explaining that in the myocardium the duration is longer than in skeletal muscle and that there is also a plateau in the myocardium.

> *"At this point, one must ask: why is the myocardial action potential so long, and why does it have a plateau, while that of skeletal muscle does not?" Gayton pg 108*

To clarify once again, the plato would be the orderly and precise meeting of these grandparents, i.e. maternal grandparents and maternal grandparents, paternal grandparents and paternal grandparents, in the potential of apathy, thus giving an annulment of apathy, which we call plato.

The author goes on to say:

> *"The heart is made up of three main types of muscle: atrial muscle, ventricular muscle and specialized excitatory and conductive fibers. The atrial and ventricular types of muscle contract* ***almost like skeletal muscles, but with a longer duration of contraction." Guyton 108***

In fact, the heart is a single muscle with several cubes, where each cube has its own autonomous function, with a great driving force that exists in no other muscle except the heart.

"Excitatory and conduction fibers, however, only contract weakly because they contain few contractile fibers, but they present automatic rhythmic electrical discharges, in the form of action potentials, or they conduct these action potentials through the heart, representing the excitatory system that controls rhythmic beats." (Guyton Pg. 07)

Excitatory fibers are not characterized by having few contractile fibers, in fact, they do not need to work with great force because their function is only conductivity, excitability, and for this reason their work has a less accelerated rhythm.

PROJECTION **OF MATER CONTRACT CELLS IN THE HEART** The same projection of these cells at work in the heart, are present in other vital organs of the body, always acting in the same way whether in the lung, kidneys, liver, skin, bone, muscles, neurons and even in nerve synapses, gas exchange or action potentials, there will be six pairs of cells there, always appearing in a block of five units or four if the parents and maternal grandparents are together.

"Each receptor is a protein complex with a total molecular weight of 275,000, the complex is composed of five protein subunits, two alpha proteins and one each of the beta, delta and gamma proteins." Guyton & Hall (Treatise on Medical Physiology, p. 88)

The author identifies that there is this group of cells, he just doesn't understand who they are; he's actually talking about Alpha, Beta, Ceci and Delta. In the heart, they are in the **(Atrial Bell)** which I'll call the 1st **atrial cube** because it's actually three cubes made up of **mater cell** leaflets. **Inside the cube**, a contraction generates pressure and it opens, generating electricity.

In the third atrial cube, we'll find the Reversal cells, Ee and Ff Hexa Mater doing the heaviest work, sending impure blood to be oxygenated.

The anatomical shape of the heart is similar to the lungs, i.e. six cubes. Both work in a closed circle, but with very different functions: one distributes blood, the other oxygenates.

"Thus, the sinus node controls the heartbeat because its frequency of

atomic discharges is higher than that of any other portion of the heart. Therefore, the sinus node is practically always the pacemaker of the normal heart." Guyton Hall (Treatise on Medical Physiology - pg. 125)

The author talks about the Alpha, Betha and Ceci cells distributed in the sinus node, which are responsible for the heartbeat, or cardiac pacemaker.

"In addition, cardiac muscle contains typical myofibrils, with actin and myosin filaments, almost identical to those found in skeletal muscles; these filaments are arranged side by side and slide together during contractions..."Guyton & Hall (Treatise on Medical Physiology, pg.)

The **"Reverse E" and "Hexa Mater"** cells are the cells that do all the work in our organism that is considered inferior, or heavy, or they are the "garrison" cells in our organism. Another important observation about these cells is that the genius of a child depends on how many maternal grandparents the child has had in its genetic formation, or in its genetic development.

DN (the reader will understand why it is called DN and not "DNA") to be a genius, needs to be contemplated from Aa to Dd, we say that the child is (Alpha Delta) or Aa-Dd. The population is almost entirely born in the letter Cc Ceci, with only one maternal grandparent who is Beta, who is always accompanied by paternal grandparents, in pairs and in the correct sequence, if, however, a fetus is contemplated with another pair of maternal grandparents, that child will be a genius. In the case of twins, only one will be given Delta grandparents, which explains why twins have different personalities. When she reaches Aa-Dd, we say that the child is Alfha. At this level, the child brings with them five thousand years of information, hence the ease with which certain children develop any skill and we say that the child is gifted, in reality the child brings millenary information ready in their brain.

Everything is involved in the conductivity process, where information is passed on to all the cells from Aa to Jj.

In the 2nd cube (No AV) or **Purkinje cube**, the left and right branches are Purkinje branches which are formed by all the parents and all the maternal grandparents. It is in these fibers that the formation of twins takes place, where the information, or rather the concession, takes place between the Mater cells from Alfha to Jj Mater Holy. Once the information has been passed on by all the maternal cells, Purkinje passes it on to the genetic code through the process of conduction via the helicases.

Attention, this concession happens first in the heart, through the Mother Cells.

The ratchet theory, and the action potential, clearly shows the performance of these cells in the organism **and the** relationship of opposing forces that are trapped in these potentials.

> *"What causes the prolonged action potential and the plateau? At this point, the question must be asked: Why is the myocardial action potential so long, and why does it present the plateau, while that of skeletal muscle is caused almost entirely by the sudden opening of a large number of so-called fast sodium channels, which allows huge numbers of sodium ions to enter the skeletal muscle fiber from the extra-cellular fluid." Guyton & Hall (Treatise on Medical Physiology pg. 108)"*

> *"In cardiac muscle, the action potential is originated by the opening of channels of two types: the same fast sodium channels as in skeletal groups, and completely different groups of slow calcium channels... " Guyton & Hall (Treatise on Medical Physiology Pg. 108, 109)*

We can see in the potential of apao, the work of the block of fathers and maternal grandmothers who represent calcium and the fathers and maternal grandmothers who represent sodium.

In the tendon chordae, in the trabeculae carneas, in the pectineus musculosae, which in reality are the actuation of the twelve contractile cells, we have these cubes that will house the mater cells always in a division similar to what has already been described and which will be shown later in this work.

In the chordae tendineae, the quartet is in the tricuspede, and looks like three cuspedes, but Aa and B, (Alfha and Beta) are together in one block, followed by Cc and Dd so they are together in this process, they are the parents and grandparents together then comes Ee and Ff is in the bicuspede, in the ventricles, the mater quartet is in the right ventricle while the garis cells are in the left ventricle doing the heaviest work which is sending oxygenated blood to the whole body.

In the lungs, the maternal cells Aa Bb Cc Dd are in the right cube and Ee Ff are in the left tubes, and are responsible for receiving oxygen, but it is sent to the capillaries by all the maternal vessels for gas exchange.

Thus, the two muscle blocks of the heart and lung always work in opposition, in antithesis, following the cardiac cycle (systole and diastole) which ends in pulmonary oxygenation or hematosis, between these two vital organs; heart and lung, thus creating a closed circle between them.

In the action potential, **potassium** is the parents and maternal grandparents; **Aa, B, D F, and calcium** are the maternal and paternal mothers; **Aa, b, c, d, e, f** and **sodium** are the parents and all the maternal and paternal grandparents; **Aa, B, C, D, E, F** but the three minerals are of fundamental importance in the acid-base balance in the organism, and contrary to what is thought about calcium, it is actually sodium that best balances the organism, because as "garrisons" of strength, it gives impulse to the contractile work. If sodium is low in the body, it's a problem for the heart.

The meeting of calcium and potassium is called plato, and note that calcium enters twice because the number of calcium is greater than potassium.

It's the meeting of maternal parents and maternal and paternal grandparents who, when they come together, give balance to the action potential or plateau. There in the lungs, all the mother cells work with oxygen and find all the maternal and paternal parents in the capillaries.

Regarding the action potentials of the myocardium, it's important to talk about the action of these five units of maternal cell pairs, where sodium is nothing more than the junction of all the maternal and paternal grandparents, Aa, B, C, D, E, F, which is why it has so much power, potassium is the junction of the fathers and maternal grandparents.

The author says that they are completely different groups and that they represent two opposite sexes. The author above asks why this action potential is so long, and why does plato exist? The author believes that it is the entry of sodium channels that causes this long potential time, but in reality the plateau would be the meeting of fathers and mothers as already explained.

The first block of maternal cells is the maximum force, there in the first two atrial tubes, the authors call the **cardiac pacemaker**, which in reality is the greatest force of the parents and two maternal grandparents; Aa, Bb, Dd together in the work called **automatism**.

The second block of cells, which are in the purkinje node, is made up of the parents and all the maternal grandparents **Aa, b, d, f.** The rest of the grandparents are the garis cells, and they take over, i.e. they do the heavy lifting when the first block of maternal cells cannot.

> *"The sinus node (also called the sinoatrial node) is a small, flattened, ellipsoid band of specialized cardiac muscle, approximately 3,000 meters wide by 15,000 meters long and 1,000 meters thick.5... The fibers of this node have almost no contractile muscle filaments and differ from the atrial muscle fibers that surround it.... However, the fibers of the sinus node connect directly to the atrial muscle fibers, so that any action potential that starts in the sinus node diffuses immediately to the wall of the atrial muscle." Guyton & Hall, (Treatise on Medical Physiology Pg.121)*

> *"At this point in what has already been discussed about the genesis and transmission of the cardiac impulse, it should be noted that the impulse normally originates in the atrial sino-node. In certain abnormal conditions this is not the case." Guyton7Hall (Treatise on Medical Physiology 123)*

> *"Some other parts of the heart can also show rhythmic intrinsic*

excitation in the same way as the fibers of the sinus node; this is particularly true for the fibers of the A-V node and those of Purkinje." Guyton & Hall (Treatise on Medical Physiology pg. 124, 125)

Now, there is no AV, there is the Purkinje cube, which begins in the 3rd atrial cube and unfolds into two branches. Purkinje is responsible for the formation of twins, but this only occurs when there is confirmation of the grandparents from Aa to Ff, just as the genius needs confirmation of the grandparents from Alfha (Aa) to Delta (Dd).

> *"The fibers of the A-V node, when not stimulated from an external site, emit intrinsic, rhythmic discharges..." Guyton & Hall Treatise on Medical Physiology pg. 125)*

In both the first and second atrial cubes and the Purkinje cube, the discharges are triggered inside the tubes, which open, sending the stimulus to the other cells.

> *"The slow conduction in the transitional, nodal and penetrating bundle A V fibers is largely explained by the reduced number of gap junctions between the successive cells of the conduction pathways, so that there is great resistance to the passage of excitatory ions from one conductive fiber to the next. In this way, it is easy to see why each cell is successively slower in its activation." Guyton & Hall (Treatise on Medical Physiology pg. 123*

In fact, the purkinje process takes place slowly, because the parents and maternal grandparents work on it. So here we present a little of the work of the Maternal Contractile Cells in the heart.

CHAPTER II

MAPPING INFORMATION ON THE FUNCTIONAL AND SCULPTURAL PATTERN OF 96 CHROMOSOMES IN GENETICS.

A new division of the strands with two strands of 12 pairs, because two chromosomes are automatically deleted at the time of ovulation, leaving 48 pairs or 46 because the father and mother are two units in one, thus forming 46 pairs of chromosomes.

In reality, there are 24 pairs of chromosomes. In this study, they act together, and always in the entire working process of the contractile mater cells.

The ribbons are being rolled up and unfolding into new ribbons, now there will be four ribbons of 12 pairs of chromosomes, then there will be four more ribbons unfolding with six pairs of chromosomes, and one last unfolding into four ribbons of three. The reader will be able to follow these unfoldings and who takes part in them a little further on.

At the beginning of this article, we talked about the movement of the **Mater Contractile Cells**, which are characterized by a control system for all the vital functions in the body.

They always work in pairs and in antithesis, or by providing feedback to the organism. It is a group of specialized, precise cells that can read up to twelve generations in pairs.

In genetics, these are 96 chromosomes or a set of maternal and paternal parents and grandparents, in chronological order and alternating between maternal and paternal, inserted into this reading, represented by the chromosomes and which gradually curl up, to unfold at the ends in a rotating chain to form new strands at first in 4 strands of 23 until they form 96 chromosomes where there will be.

It is a rational team that is responsible for the entire process of cellular reproduction; it is characterized by forming a group of generations that reaches an average of 1000 years in each individual. This explains why certain children give us the impression that they were born knowing a lot, especially the AaDd, Alfha Delta, children who can play the piano at a very early age, or can count, or have a fantastic memory, or even speak a foreign language without any effort, and that in reality, each of us brings a hundred generations into our presence.

Our genetic code gives us a correct third and even fourth generation record for the Alpha Delta; therefore, we need to be aware of what we are producing as human beings, what values we are passing on to our future generations, how we are experiencing humanitarian ethics, because these generations are the ones who control and reproduce the next generations. Or rather, each one of us will be present in our descendants for approximately a thousand years. We can influence our ethical and moral values for up to a thousand years, everything is impregnated in our cellular system.

Don't forget that. That's why it's important that we improve as human beings, otherwise we could found a sick society, or a highly intelligent one over the years, driven only by the commands of our cellular system.

We can observe this by looking at the Jews, Japanese, Germans, Chinese, etc. All the knowledge acquired over the generations is passed on through the DN. If we don't improve as human beings, LUPUS will be a growing disease, along with cancer and other diseases, especially rheumatological and neurological diseases, especially headache, which will fill all existing hospitals, clinics and consultancies.

Authors, whether in genetics or physiology, say that genes control cell function, the substances to be used, structure, enzymes, etc. There is a lot to explain in this study, but from everything we already know, the maternal contractile cells are responsible for controlling everything related to the new being.

Therefore, all this work belongs to the **maternal contractile cells**, which go beyond these functions, they determine genetics, from sex to skin color, eyes, hair, gifts, luck and even wealth, genius and quantity,everything will depend exclusively on the representation of the hereditary set present in each genetic reproduction, formed by a hundred maternal and paternal mothers with a representation at the end of six pairs of chromosomes that is the genetic skeleton, where the **genetic code, the gene, the DN** will be specified, but they are the same characters in all cells

Mater in the rest of the organism; parents and grandparents always in pairs, or only the grandparents together, or only the grandparents together, depending on where they work, or the role they play.

All decisions are made automatically, through chemical processes within the board of this Celulas Contrateis Mater team. Nothing is random, they are chemical processes, but there is a decision that needs to be made very quickly and precisely between the members.

Guyton and Hall say:

> *"Almost everyone knows that genes, located in the nuclei of every cell in the body, control heredity from parents to children, but most people don't realize that even these genes also control the functioning of every cell in the body. Genes control cell function, determining which substances are synthesized by the cell, which structures, which enzymes, which chemicals." (Guyton and Hall pg.27)*

> *"Each gene, which is the nucleic acid called deoxyribonucleic acid (DNA), automatically controls the formation of another acid, called ribonucleic acid (RNA), which spreads from the cell and controls the formation of a specific protein." (Guyton and Hall p.27)*

The gene could never be an acid because, according to this study, genes are made up exclusively of QB base group moieties which are deoxyribose, i.e. oxygen. Then there is no such thing as DNA, firstly because it is not an acid. DN is also made up of QB moieties and they are oxygen, and DN is also made up of a cube, which we can call the DN cube, where not information is stored, but the genetic inheritance of generations and never of diseases. The rest of the information is in the genetic code. If you've read what we've written before, you can see how the sentences in these texts make no sense. The gene contains acid, but the DN is not an acid nor is the RN an acid, in genetics the command is of the QB women and they do not have acid, they only have oxygen, the men, who are part of the **"nitrogenous base and phosphoric acid".**

This study will map out the behavior of chromosomes, who they really are, and what they do, i.e. the specific function of each of them, so that the reader will understand when the inaccurate contents that appear in the texts are clarified, due to the authors' lack of knowledge about who really acts in a DN, in an RN, in the genetic code, etc.

Let's see, what Guyton says in the text mentioned above, that all the genes are in the nucleus of all the cells, controlling the functioning of all the cells.

Genes are the specific merits of a few rare fertilizations, because gene in genetics refers to the genius of a child, and of course the genealogical tree is involved in all this, because the AaDd brings the genealogy of four generations in pairs together.

It can't be in every cell because, to be a gene, it needs to meet certain criteria: it needs to be similar between two maternal grandparents and the paternal grandparents, so the genes belong to the Alpha Delta. Guyton then goes on to say that the gene is the deoxyribonucleic nucleic acid.

Acid, only women work in the DN, acid and when it acts only men, and also it does not control the RN, on the contrary, the RN has the function of transcribing the contents of the chromosomes, informing if there are genes for the Ribosomes. Those who control heredity are the coronary genes, which send their commands through the conduction process: Alpha, Beta, Ceci, Delta, Reverse E, Hexa Mater. The genes also control how many babies will be born, this is done through the Purkinje fibers.

CHROMOSOME STRAND UNFOLDING FOR GENE CODING

First Tape - (Nitro Tape)
Aa-Bb-Cc-Ee-Gg-Ii

Second Tape

In this second strand we have the Nucleotides with 24 pairs of chromosomes, so we have the second unfolding, then a new unfolding in 12 pairs of chromosomes which is formed by the paternal grandparents and are the acids, and the **Nitrogenous Base** which is the only time the acids appear. They are **(Aa- C- E-G-I-L-N-P-R-T-V-Z).**

Genetics works more with oxygen, which is the maternal grandparents who make most of the commands, including DN.

After this unfolding, this strand is left with six pairs of chromosomes **(Aa- Cc-Ee-Gg-Ii-Ll), which** are the **phosphoric acids** and send the reading to the second strand, which then unfolds into three pairs of chromosomes formed by an acid-only base, **the Helicases (Aa-Cc_-Ee-)**, which send this result to the base. On this strand we refer to the acids which are: **Nitrogenous Base** and **Phosphoric Acid and Helicases.**

Third Tape, QB - (I want it good)

It is now made up of all the maternal grandparents, who are **RN- Aa-B(b)-D(d)-F(f)-H(h)-J(j)-M(m)-O(o)-Q(q)-S(s)-U(u)-X(x),** reads the first strand and sends the results of the **genetic transcription** to the third strand. After sending the transcriptions of the two strands together, this second strand makes a new split into six pairs of chromosomes, or **Transcription (Aa-Bb-Dd-Ff-Hh-Jj)** and then makes a new split into just three pairs of chromosomes or **DN (Aa-Bb-Dd)** We speak of this strand as **RN Transcription and DN.**

The Fourth Strand (Deoxyribose Strand)

It is formed by the parents and twelve maternal grandparents who are the Aa b- d- f-h-j-m-o-q-s-u-x **Ribosomes**. This strand receives the information from the three strands together and sends the transcript to the fourth strand. It then unfolds again into six pairs of chromosomes which are the **Deoxyribose (Aa-Bb-Dd-Ff-Hh-Jj)** which are maternal mothers. This is followed by a further split into three pairs of chromosomes, **which** are the **Enzymes (Aa-Bb-Dd).** Here we talk about **Ribosomes and Deoxyribose** Enzymes to make it easier for the authors to study.

The fifth tape (TRIPE)

It is a kit of twelve generations of maternal grandparents; Aa-B(b)-D(d)-F(f)-H(h)-J(j) (M)m (O)o (Q)q-(S)s-(U)u-(X)x and a final reading of the three previous tapes is made to form the **genetic skeleton** (Aa-Bb-Cc-Dd-Ee-Ff).

The **Genetic Code** is not the same thing as the **DN**, the latter is the nucleus of the cell and is formed strictly by QB mothers and the genetic code shows the generations contained in the genetic skeleton, these are generations in each individual that reach about five thousand years. But we are left with only twelve generations, six of which are active and present; the rest could be harmful to our organism. **Eversion (Ee**) gets its name because this cell in other organs can already be harmful in its actions. In Genetics, this risk occurs from Mm onwards.

The Genetic Code is formed by the parents and grandparents **QB (Aa-Bb-Dd-Ff),** which means that they will always be faithful to the genetic skeleton without trying to destroy it, since an intense battle takes place until the skeleton is formed, many pairs of chromosomes will become harmful and try to destroy the fertilized ovum, an example of which are congenital deformities, mutilations and so we have a huge list of these results.

Pay attention to some important information; Gene refers only to genius offspring, those with two consecutive maternal grandparents, Bb and Dd, or the direct inheritance of eight genealogical trees. The Gene has its direct command from the heart, through the process of conduction.

From the letter Mm onwards, these chromosomes are antigens in our organism, they try to destroy the first chromosomes, and cause mutations, especially if it's a gene, if it's twins, then they try to deform, mutilate etc. One example is Down's syndrome. DN controls and determines the death of these cells, which are harmful to the organism from Mm onwards. Mothers are up to Jj and fathers up to Ll.

MAPPING AND FUNCTIONAL MODELING OF CHROMOSOMES IN GENETICS

Before we start the mapping, remember that in genetics, maternal grandparents are present in almost every classification, the grandparents are the acids and have a single weight, as will be shown.

1- **Phosphoric acid** is formed by the paternal grandparents: (A)a-(B)b-(C)c-(E)e(G)g-(I)i- (L)l

2- **Deoxyribose-** They are six maternal avos A(a)- B(b)- D(d)-F(f)-H(h)-J(j)

3- **Nitrogenous base-** All paternal grandparents: Aa-(C)c- (E)e-(G)g- (I)i- (L)l-(N)n-(P)p-(R)r-(T)t-(V)v-(Z)z.

4- **The nucleotides** are the parents and all the maternal and paternal grandparents together Aa-Bb-Cc-Dd-Ee-Ff-Gg-Hh-Ii-Jj-Ll-Mm-Nn-Oo-Pp-Qq-Rr-Ss-Tt-Uu-Vv-Xx-Zz.

5- **The skeleton of the DN is** formed by the parents and maternal grandparents:

Alfha Mater (Aa)
Beta (Bb)
Delta (Dd)
Hexa Mater (Ff
Mater Holey H (Hh)
Jota Holey (Jj)

6- **The nucleus of the DN** is formed by the parents, and the maternal grandparents

Alfha (AaBb)
Delta (Dd)
Hexa Mater (Ff)

Attention: in this cube we have AaBb which are joined together.

7- **The RN** is formed by the parents Alfha Mater and all the grandparents together in sequence in a ribbon of twelve, Aa- Bb-Dd -FF-HH-JJ-Mm-OO-Qq-SS-Uu-Xx .

8- **Transcription -** It's actually a kind of bookcase with folders on all hereditary genetics. It's a summary of all the parents and maternal grandparents (QB) from Aa to Jj, where the QB (I mean well) Aa-Bb -Dd-Ff- Hh-Jj is contained.

9- **DN Polymerase** does not exist and the same DN (Alpha (Aa) Beta (Bb) Delta (Dd)) (Ff)

10- **The Triplets (TRIPE)**, because they read three consecutive tapes, are a kit of twelve generations of consecutive maternal grandparents, together with the parents who recognize these generations and send this reading to the base, until the skeleton is formed. Aa-Bb-Dd-Ff-Hh-Jj-Mm-OO-Qq-SS-Uu-Xx

11- **The chromosomes** are all the grandparents together, maternal and paternal, making a total of 100 in the sequence or 50 pairs.

12- Enzymes are the three mothers: ALFHA -BETA - DELTA

13- **Helicase-** are all the mater QB avos: Aa- (B)b-(D)d.

14- **Ribosomes** are all maternal grandparents- Aa-b-d-f-h-j-m-o-q-s-u-x

15- **The genetic code-** is only the grandparents QB- AaBb- Cc-Dd. The genetic code is directly related to the heart.

Other codifications to facilitate this study:

Purine is an acid base: Aa-C-E-G-I-L

Guanine: C-E

Perimidinic and a deoxy base They are: Aa-b-d

Cytosine- Aa-b-d-f

SUMMARY of the tapes

First tape splitting base for encoding

Chromosomes - 96 Consecutive maternal and paternal fathers and mothers together

Nucleotides - These are the 23 pairs of chromosomes together on the same strand, maternal and paternal grandparents.

Nitrogenous base - All the paternal grandparents together. 12 pairs of chromosomes

RN- All maternal grandparents together, 12 pairs

Ribosomes - 12 maternal grandparents together

TRIPE - 12 maternal grandparents together

Second tape splitting base for encoding

Phosphoric Acid - The paternal grandparents 6 pairs of Chromosomes

Transcription - with six pairs of chromosomes

Deoxyribose- with six pairs of chromosomes.

DN skeleton - with six pairs of chromosomes

The third tape deployment base

Helicases, with three pairs of chromosomes

DN- With three pairs of chromosomes. Attenuation AaBb form a single Dd-Ff unit.

Enzymes with three pairs of chromosomes

Genetic code with three pairs of chromosomes

So we can conclude that nucleotides are made up of four coiled strands of six chromosomes each, where they end up in the skeleton to transcribe the genetic code.

Guyton goes on to say that "DNA automatically controls another acid, which is RNA."

NBs cannot be acidic because they are formed by mothers and, in the same way as NBs are formed by maternal grandmothers, they are gases formed by oxygen, and it is they who take care of the gas exchange process in the lungs.

Says the author:

> *" The human body has thousands of control systems. The most intricate of these is the genetic control system that operates in every cell to control intra- and extra-cellular functions.... Others operate throughout the body to control the interplay between organs." Guyton & Hall pg. 06*

The human body has only one type of control and that is the Mater contractile cells, and the same system operates in genetics, neurology, cardiology, physiology, respiratory, only in genetics, the system changes a lot because instead of dealing with six Mater cells, twelve generations of Mater cells are used and furthermore there are 24 members of these cells instead of six.

It is here that we show a little of the work of the waste disposal in the reproductive system, these cells work in a special, careful, coherent way, as has already been explained, carefully reading the generations, working in a precise, cautious, fair way, reading and re-reading everything that is done, nothing can go wrong, and when it comes to fines, are those pairs of grandparents at the end of the tape, which are already reversed to the organism and concomitantly to the fetus, and these are dirtying the organization of the work of the other group of deoxyribose cells and this is how the anomalies are happening are the same pair of grandparents of Dawn syndrome, this one has no more commitment to the lineage, and is at the end of the tape as reversed cells, so, the errors in the fines are not errors on the part of the triplets, who are the readers, and they are precise, and the action of the cosmic dust or Lixo Sitiante, which are reverse cell commands, is what is also being addressed in this study, not to mention that in this system, an immense battle is fought, because there are 24 maternal and paternal grandparents who stand in an assembly position and all give their opinion on the characteristics of the offspring, But be careful, the only ones who give their opinion on genius, physical characteristics and duplicity are the six closest, that is, from Aa to Ff. They all have to agree that the child is a twin, or on the color of the skin of the eyes, or on the fact that the child is a genius. Regarding physical characteristics, the inheritance will only be from the parents, (Alfha) and the first maternal grandparents (Bb) Beta and the paternal grandparents (Cc) Ceci, unless the child is Aa-Dd...

All opinions are given in descending order, with the greatest being the parents (Alfha), followed by the maternal grandparents and paternal grandparents and so on, in a course of twelve generations, with twelve grandparents on one side and twelve on the other. Everything that belongs to the child is passed on between all the grandparents, who may or may not allow what is established.

There is a criterion for who can have the strongest opinion, for who can decide on the characteristics of the child, and each member of the genetic Mater cell obeys these criteria, the maternal grandparents or the "triplets" are in charge of all this, and they are the ones who read about the hundred maternal and paternal mothers and pass this information on to the base and in the end these generations are deleted, leaving only the essential genetic base from Aa to Ff.

The parents and three maternal grandparents and two paternal grandparents in pairs. It needs to be careful, coherent, precise, it involves more human mater cells which are all the rest of the genetic inheritance that is a total of twelve maternal grandparents where the quartet always appears; the parents and two maternal grandparents and the parents or Alfha Mater are two in one so we have 24 pairs for a total of 48 chromosomes.

Thus, genetic work is differentiated from other functional systems in our organism, since it includes all Mater and Pater cells.

"The importance of DNA lies in its ability to control the formation of proteins by the cell. It does this through the genetic code."

"The genetic code consists of successive "triplets" of bases - that is, each successive three bases is a word of the code. It can be seen that these triplets are respectively responsible for the successive insertion of the three amino acids - proline, serine and glutamic acid.

The triplets or TRIPE are actually the maternal grandparents, recognizing up to one hundred mothers or maternal grandparents, and sending this reading to the base for encoding.

> *"Because DNA is located in the nucleus of the cell, while most of the cell's functions are carried out in the cytoplasm, there must be some way in which the genes in the nucleus control the chemical reactions in the cytoplasm. This involves the intermediation of another type of nucleic acid, RNA, whose formation is controlled by the nucleus' DNA. Guyton & Hall pg. 29*

The chemical reactions are controlled by the DN, which is transcribed by the RN and transformed into enzymes to encode all the information contained in the fertilized egg.

> *"As with all important events in the cell, reproduction begins in the nucleus itself. The first step is the replication of all the DNA in the chromosomes, only after which mitosis can take place." Guyton & Hall pg.3*

> *"The human cell contains 46 chromosomes arranged in 23 pairs. In a pair, most of the genes on one chromosome are identical, or almost identical, to the genes on the other chromosome, so it can generally be said that genes exist in pairs, although this is not always the case." Guyton & Hall pg.38*

The author says that genes are identical and do not always appear in pairs, they are identical, and always work in pairs, this can in no way be changed, unless there is an action of the Besieging Trash on the cells, in which case, as has already been informed, we will have mutations.

> *"During the hour or so between DNA replication and the start of mitosis, there is a period of very active repair and proof-reading of the DNA strands, where inappropriate nucleotides have been paired with nucleotides from the original template strand, special enzymes cut out*

the defective areas and replace them with completely appropriate nucleotides.... As a result of the repair of this proof reading, the transcription process rarely makes mistakes, when there is a mistake there is a mutation. Guyton & Hall pg. 28

It takes exactly one hour for each baby or for each gene to start mitosis, and there are no inappropriate or defective nucleotides whatsoever, and there is an exact number of cells that must remain and that must leave.

Everything is done with precision and when the mutation occurs then we already have another process involved, which would be the garbage settling on the cell. Everything is done very quickly because there is a great fear that the egg cells will be destroyed by the last paternal grandparents, they are already against it, so everything has to be decided quickly, and watch out, the permissiveness of everything will reach the letter Ff.

SELF REPLICATION - "THE PRINCIPLE OF PARELING"

"According to the pentose they contain, nucleic acids are of two types: DNA (deoxyribonucleic acid) which contains deoxyribose, and RNA (ribonucleic acid) which contains ribose." (Borges Osorio, mª Regina, 2001 p.20)

"The code for the production of the different types of proteins that the organism must make throughout its life is contained in the egg cell of each individual. All the cells of a given organism, at a given moment in their life, contain the same code or genetic information as that first cell. However, not all genes are functioning in all cells at the same time and with the same intensity. This varies with the type of cell and the age of the individual". (Borges Osorio, MF Regina, 2001 p. 20)

Each gene receives its coding through a joint, specialized, precise work between its pairs of chromosomes where everything is carefully read, interpreted and coded without errors and following patterns of genetic heredity, but there is no disease in these codes or in these egg cells, of characteristics coded in the genes by hereditary order.

Attention, there are no genes working in the cells, what exists is a joint work in an organized, precise team acting in all the egg cells in the fertilization process.

The egg cell is formed by a genetic code made up of the parents, Aa (Alpha Mater) Bb (Beta Mater) Cc- (Ceci) Dd (Delta) . They always obey a specific order, in ascending order, alternating as shown above, thus ending their genetic inheritance in each individual.

The proteins involved in the formation of each gene, the helices, are batches of this information that do not mix, they are independent even though they come together, as has already been explained, and the first maternal grandparent is the one most involved in the formation of the child's genes.

Therefore, genes do not vary according to the age of the individual, they come specified and face a great battle with the junk (this study is in another work by the same authors) to remain perfect in their base, but they are often mutated, so it is not the code that is inherited from mutations by the mother or grandmother, the mutations or deformations are the result of a battle fought between these chromosomes before they are deleted. Everything is done quickly and precisely, but they are still attacked by other chromosomes that are harmful to the organism before they die. The QB grandparents always try to defend the egg during fertilization, but the results are not always positive, but there are no errors or deforming heredity.

> *"The genetic code describes the relationship between the sequence of nitrogenous bases and the sequence of amino acids and forms the unit of genetic information or codon." (Borges- Osorio, MF Machado, 2001 p. 22)*

"Its reading is done on nucleic base cracks".

The reading is done individually on each gene, although they are together.

DN TYPES

DN Nuclear

Non-repetitive DNA, according to the author:

> *"the distribution of these genes varies greatly between the different chromosomes and in certain chromosomal regions"*

The destruction is of the Reverse chromosomes, as explained above.

Moderately repetitive DNA

> *"It consists of a small number of copies per genome, containing multigenic families"...(Borges Osorio and Mª Regina p. 25)*

There is no small number of copies per genome, but a sequential, equal and perfect reconnection with the participation of all the maternal grandparents who are directly responsible for this coding.

There are variations simply due to the entry of LS into the cell, which ends up modifying its function, which is where the mutilations originate.

The distribution of genes is equal and perfect, with no variation.

Highly repetitive DNA

> *"There are genes that are similar to structural genes, but which are not functionally expressed. These genes are called pseudogenes and appear to have arisen through duplication and the acquisition of many mutations in the coding and regulatory elements..." (Borges Osorio and M³ Regina p. 25)*

Regarding these identical genes, they have not arisen through duplication and even less through the acquisition of many mutations. What happens is an organized process, where forces are measured, weighed and discussed in an assembly with a small population of 24 chromosomes.

When we have the same problem in a particular family, we don't have a genetic inheritance, but a deforming genetics caused by external factors such as garbage.

mitochondrial DNA according to the author:

> *"It is a circular double-stranded DNA found inside mitochondria, energy-producing organelles located inside the cytoplasm of practically all eukaryotic cells. This DNA has no crossing-over, no histone frameworks, no repair system, practically exists in many copies per mitochondrion and per cell, is maternally inherited and is highly exposed to free oxygen radicals." (Borges Osorio and M Regina p. 25)*
>
> *"Eukaryotic cells contain a variable number of mitochondria, depending on the energy needed to carry out their functions; the greater this need, as in muscles and the brain, for example, the greater the amount of mitochondria in the cell cytoplasm." (Borges Osorio and Mª Regina p. 26)*

The mitochondria are the QB grandparents, there are a total of six, Aa-b-d-f, which in genetics are what define whether the fertilized egg will be a female or a double female, they are energy carriers, because they have the gases hydrogen, nitrogen, and are responsible for this work of double chain circulation, but there are multiple copies per mitochondria, which will be the formation of twins.

Just as there is no system of repair and crossing-over, because when genes are formed, the genes are coded perfectly in pairs, starting with the maternal parents and ending with the paternal parents.

The author says: *"Thus, a disease caused by a mutation in the mt DNA is inherited exclusively from the mother. Therefore, only women can transmit mitochondrial diseases, passing on the mutations to all their offspring of both sexes. However, this transmission does not seem so simple, because the expression of some mitochondrial genes depends on interaction with nuclear genes, the mechanism of which is obscure, given that mt DNA replicates independently of nuclear DNA" (Borges Osorio and Mª Regina p. 28).*

Now, it's not true that women transmit mitochondrial diseases, what happens is the LS inside the cell, this garbage can come from the Reverse cells that can do this, that is, try to destroy a coding because it doesn't accept it, or it can come from afferent commands. The only cells that don't lend themselves to this role are the Aa-Bb-Dd-Ff maternal cells, nor is it true that the expression of some mitochondrial genes depends on interaction with nuclear genes, which is why the author says that this mechanism is still obscure. DN is always carried out flawlessly and with accurate genetic data, but it can already be altered by LS at the time of replication.

The author goes on to say:

> *"Therefore, mitochondrial diseases are most often characterized by myopathies and encephalopathies, problems in the muscles and brain respectively. Finally, oxidative phosphorylation declines with age, perhaps due to the accumulation of mutations in mtDNA. Thus, the clinical phenotype in mitochondrial diseases (such as Leber's hereditary optic neuropathy, hypertrophic cardiomyopathy with myopathy and maternally inherited diabetes with deafness) is not directly related to the mtDNA genotype, but reflects various factors such as those already mentioned." Apub pg. 28*

The mitochondria are great carriers of sedentary waste, as has already been said in this study, they contain the oxygen that the waste needs to be carried, so the mitochondria in a way end up being largely responsible for mitochondrial diseases. Now, phosphorylation doesn't decline with age, but with sedentarization, in mitochondria, which are themselves a real depository of LS.

HEREDITARY METABOLIC ERRORS

Says the author:

"Inherited metabolic errors are genetically determined biochemical disorders in which a specific enzyme defect produces a metabolic blockage that can lead to a disease." Apub pb. 29

Enzymes can't give rise to diseases because, according to our table, they are the parents and the first two maternal grandparents.

"At the moment of replication, these bonds break and the double helix opens with the help of enzymes called helicases, leaving its ends free to bind to new specific nucleotides. Each strand directs and serves as a template for the synthesis of a new strand by complementary base pairing, from nucleotides present in the cell nucleus." Guyton & Hall PG. 31

"The principle of complementary base pairing states that an unpaired base attracts a free nucleotide only if it is complementary." Guyton & Hall PG. 31

The double helices don't open with the help of enzymes, each strand has its own job to do and they act as a community, where each cell has its own role to play. It has already been said in this study that there are no specific nucleotides, nor is it true that one new filament serves as a template for another, one unfolds into the other, but there is a goal, they gradually loosen until they reach the nucleus of the cell.

Nor is it true that one unpaired base attracts another; what happens is that the nucleotides unfold until they reach the skeleton for transcription.

In the terminals six Mater cells bind to new specific nucleotides and it is not a new filament, but the set of all Mater cells that form a base from the nucleotide present in the cell's nucleus.

Says author Guyton:

"The nucleotides link together to form the two DN strands. They are loosely bound together by weak cross-links. The skeleton of each DN is

composed of alternating molecules of phosphoric acid and deoxyribose. The purine and pyrimidine bases are attached to the sides of the deoxyribose molecules. The two strands of DNA are held together by a hydrogen bridge." Apub pg. 32

The DN is composed of the QB mothers (I mean well) so they are Aa-Bb-Dd, the purine bases are therefore alterations of phosphoric acid and deoxyribose molecules and the pyrimidine bases are attached to the sides.

The RNs are assembled under the influence of enzymes called RN polymerase. The two strands are actually four strands of six chromosomes forming nucleotides that unfold until they reach the genetic code.

According to Guyton:

Each strand's purine adenine base always joins the other strand's pyrimidine thymine base.

They are natural unfoldings from one base to another.

Each base decides on the gene, if it's a man, where the characteristics come from, everything needs to be resolved very quickly, because the gene could be destroyed.

The Gene decision is made following other criteria within each base.

Each guanine purine base always joins the cytosine pyrimidine base.

Attention: Purinic Guanine- Aa- Cc- Ee-Gg-Ii-Ll are the nitrogenous acid base. Pyrimidine Cytosine- These are the oxygenated base or deoxyribose. That's why one base always joins the other, meaning that the nitrogenous base or the male always joins the oxygenated base or the female and confirms that we are duplicates or twins.

Assembly of the RNA chain with the activated nucleotides using the DNA strand as a template.

If you look at what has been written about the coding bases, you'll find this answer, because the RN receives the reading of the nitrogenous base and sends the transcription of the two bases to a third base, the Ribosomes.

The RNA molecule is assembled under the influence of the enzyme RNA polymerase. This is a large protein that has many of the functional properties necessary for the formation of the RNA molecule: In the DNA strand at the beginning of each gene, there is a sequence of nucleotides called a promoter. RNA polymerase has an appropriate complementary structure, which recognizes this promoter and binds to it. This is the essential step to start the formation of RNA molecules.

After binding to the promoter, RNA polymerase causes about two turns of the DNA helix to unwind and the two strands to separate in the unwound region.

The reader should note what has been written about this item previously, as the split happens directly between RN and DN with all the transcription of heredity.

The polymerase then moves along the DNA strand, temporarily unwinding and separating the two DN strands at each stage of its movement

What happens is that RN unfolds into DN, leading to its transcription, on the nitrogenous base, so that the strands unfold.

First it forms the hydrogen bridge between the next base in the DNA strand and the base of the RNA nucleotide

The polymerase then cleaves two or three phosphates from each of the RNA nucleotides, releasing a large amount of energy from the phosphate bonds. This energy is used to form the covalent bond between the remaining phosphate in the niclotide and the ribose at the end of the RNA chain being formed.

When the RNA polymerase reaches the end of the DNA gene, it encounters a new DN A nucleotide sequence called the chain termination sequence.

This causes the polymerase and the newly formed DNA strand to separate from the DN strand. The polymerase can then be reused successively to form other RNA strands.

Attention, there is no polymerase and DNA chain separating from DN, it all means the same thing, a strand of RN transcribes to DN and ends in DN.

As the new RNA strand is formed, the weak hydrogen bridges with the DNA strand are broken, as the DNA has a high affinity for binding to the complementary DNA strand. Thus, the RNA chain detaches from the DN and is released into the nucleoplasm. In this way, the code present in the DNA strand is transmitted in a complementary way to the RNA strand. The ribose nucleotide bases always combine with the deoxyribose bases as follows in the unfolding.

Attention: Nucleotides are not functional bases, they are only present in the first unfolding, and it is the nitrogenous base for men that combines with the deoxyribose base for women, so this combination is fair.

All the explanations about the unfolding of the chromosomes are translated in this study, where the author can see how everything is very simple and clear, there are no complications, and any student of the subject can easily understand this study.

FOUR DIFFERENT TYPES OF RNA.

Messenger RNA - which carries the genetic code to the cytoplasm to control the type of protein formed.

Transfer RNA that transports the activated amino acids to the ribosomes, the amino acids will be used to assemble the protein molecule.

Ribosomal RNA which, with around 75 different proteins, forms ribosomes, the physical and chemical structures in which protein molecules are formed.

Micro RNA - which are single-stranded RNA molecules of 21 to 23 nucleotides that regulate gene transcription and translation.

According to what has already been written in this study, the RN has only three functions and no more. It receives all the readings from the nitrogenous base, sends this information to the DN and unfolds 12 pairs of chromosomes into six pairs of chromosomes which are the DN, then transcribes the readings to the next base which are the ribosomes and completes all its functions in genetics.

Everything that has been said about the organization of nucleotides is summed up in their unfolding, which gradually loosens their strands until they reach the desired number for coding the gene with the three main QB mothers Aa-Bb-Cc- Dd.

CHAPTER III

IMMUNE SYSTEM - IMMUNITY BLOCK

In the Immune System, we once again have the organization of the Mater Contractile cells, working together in the "deoxyribose" block of immunity, but we will encounter the action of the reverse cells that try to destroy the Q/B base group.

> *"The term immunity is derived from the Latin word immunitas, which refers to the protection against legal proceedings that Roman senators had during their term of office." Abul K. Abbas-Andrew H. Lichtman pg .03*

The term immunity, therefore, was already used in ancient Rome, when Roman citizens who were elected senators were guaranteed protection against legal proceedings during their term of office. In the course of history, this term was transferred to health as protection against infectious diseases. Mater cells are also responsible for immunity in the body, forming the immune system.

> *"The cells and molecules responsible for immunity form the immune system, and their collective and coordinated response to the introduction of foreign substances is called the immune response." Apud pg. 3*

> *"The physiological function of the immune system is defense against infectious microorganisms." Abul K. Abbas and Andrew H. Lichtman pg. 03 text General properties of immune responses.*

This study brings a new concept to this system, by understanding that the immune system is characterized by the rivalry between two groups of cells: on the one hand, the Mater Cells, of the Q/B group, and on the other, the Reverse Cells, or even the nitrous acids against the basic Q/B.

Nitro Acids- Aa-Cc-Ee-Gg-Ii-Ll-Nn-Pp-Rr-Tt-Vv-Zz

Mother Cells- Aa-Bb-Dd-Ff-Hh-Jj-Mm-Oo-Qq-Ss-Uu-Uu-Xx

MACROPHAGES, OUR BIGGEST ENEMY IN THE IMMUNE SYSTEM

Everything that has been written to date about the immune system does not correspond to the reality of the facts; The Immune System is a system that can be compared to our real world, where there is a rivalry between two groups of cells. On the one hand, the Mater cell group tries to remove foreign substances from the organism, to rid it of infections, but the Reverse group, formed by macrophages, tries to destroy these protective cells at all costs, targeting the Alpha Memory cells, which are the antigens that are distinguished from the others by their highly trained memory.

Macrophages use perversity, in short, they fight an immense battle with defined targets, just like in a war. If you're looking for the enemy, you use strategies to capture it.

MAIN COMPONENTS OF THE IMMUNE SYSTEM

In the Immune system we will find the same components that we have already studied in genetics, the difference is that in genetics, all the time we had the action of deoxyribose, that is the mothers, in the Immune system, we will find the action of acids in search of Alpha Memory.

We'll give an overview of the components found in the immune system, then we'll map them out so that the reader can better understand the functionality of the events that appear in the immune system and realize that the concepts put forward by all the authors who have studied this subject have failed to understand how this system works.

Let's take, for example, what the authors say about antigens:

> *"Foreign substances that induce specific immunological responses or are the target of such responses. If they develop before invasion by microorganisms, they must have some mechanism for recognizing that invasion." Abul K. Abbas and Andrew H. Lichtman pg. 03*

In cardiology, the authors of this study explained that maternal contractile cells are present throughout the body, developing all vital functions. The immune system is no different: the antigens or "genos" are the maternal parents and grandparents of Alpha Memory (Aa-Bb-Dd-Ff-Hh-Jj-Mm-), therefore they are extremely important in the immune system, but they are constant targets for phagocytosis by macrophages, mainly because these antigens are part of the group.

Alfha-Delta, which are insensitively sought after in the body, have an extraordinary memory, so antigens are by no means elements that come to destroy our organism, as well as other components that are more in a position to defend our organism.

Components of the immune system

Basic Q/B group

1- Lymphocytes - Alpha-Delta (Aa-Bb-Dd) and Alpha-Ceci (Aa-Bb-Cc)

2- Antigens -Alfha-memory (Aa-Bb-Dd-Ff-Hh-Jj-Mm) Maternal grandparents

3- Eosinophils-Alfha-Son (Aa-Bb-Dd-Ff-Hh-Jj-Mm-Oo-Qq-Ss) (They are characterized by being good throughout their existence, they are like that because they were born in a high human HR score They are grandparents who were good children)

4- Antibodies are the entire deoxyribose line from Alpha to Mater Son. Aa-Bb-Dd-Ff-Hh-Jj-Mm-Oo-Qq-Ss, so they are Alpha-son radars because they work exactly like radars in the immune system, looking for particles that are harmful to the body.

Reversa Group

1-Macrophages (Aa-Bb-Cc-Ee-Gg-Ii-Ll-Nn-Pp-Rr-Tt-Vv-Zz) Although the ribbon appears complete, macrophages are exactly the reverse cells (Rr-Tt-Vv-Zz). They are therefore the last cells that are no longer part of the QB group, they are totally harmful to the organism, and highly destructive.

In the formation of the fetus, these letters are the ones that cause deformities in the fetus affecting several generations, which is why it gives the impression that certain diseases that pass from one generation to another are hereditary, but in reality, it would be the same pair of chromosomes, represented by the grandparents as has already been explained, that does this work of destroying the fetus in some generations.

PROPERTIES OF THE IMMUNE RESPONSE

There are only three types of immunity:

Natural Immunity - formed by the lymphocytes that are represented by the parents and maternal and paternal grandparents (Alfha- Ceci) (Aa- Bb-Cc)
Acquired Immunity - Formed by Antigens - These are all the avos of the basic Q/B group, i.e. all the good Alfha-Memory avos(Aa-Bb- Dd-Ff-Hh-Jj-Mm-)
Adaptive Immunity - Formed by Eosinophils - They are represented by all the good grandparents, they are the last ones on the ribbon that help the Immune System when everything has been tried, an example would be Lupus. Alfha Son (Aa-Bb-Dd-Ff-Hh-Jj-Mm-Oo-Qq-Ss)

NATURAL IMMUNITY:

Natural immunity is immunity that is pre-established in the body, i.e. the person is born with it. In the immune system, the group of maternal cells responsible for immunity are the lymphocytes (Aa-Bb-Cc), which are made up exclusively of parents and maternal grandparents.

They take care of re-establishing the body's existing immunity at the first moment it is needed, an example would be a cut, at the same moment as the accident occurs, the cut appears with phlogistic signs, above all from the cytokines which are the maternal grandparents, six pairs of grandparents act here. It is they, or rather they, who cause vasodilation, the fathers and maternal grandfathers (prostaglandin plus bradykinin), who cause the smooth muscle of the vessels to relax, thus allowing more blood to flow and facilitating the help of the Alfha- Memory.

> *"Natural immunity consists of cellular and biochemical defense mechanisms that already existed before the establishment of an infection, and that are programmed to respond quickly to an infection." Abul K. Abbas pg4*
>
> *"The main components of the natural Immune System are: 1-physical and chemical barriers, such as the epithelium and antibacterial substances on the epithelial surfaces, 2-neutrophil and macrophage phagocytic cells...." Abul K. Abbas pg4*

Firstly, there are no barriers or biochemical defense mechanisms in the natural system, it is in fact the parents and maternal grandparents who take care of the defense of the organism, then the phagocytic cells, especially the macrophages, are in no way part of the natural system, and then the neutrophils, which are part of the basic Q/B group with a specific type of immunological defense.

Natural immunity consists of

B-lymphocytes - Alpha-Delta- (Aa-Bb-Cc-Dd) These are the fathers and maternal grandfathers.

Alpha-memory T-lymphocytes (Aa-Bb-Cc-Dd-Ff-Hh-Jj-Mm) are the parents and paternal grandparents of the Q/B group.

ACQUIRED IMMUNITY: ANTIGENS (ALFHA-HOLY JOTA)

The immune system works in blocks, so antigens are part of acquired immunity because they are constantly requested by the Alpha-Son and Alpha-Delta lymphocytes to inform them of the type of invader that has arrived in the body and what substance it contains so that it can be phagocytosed. Antigens communicate with antibodies via their receptors, which are made up of the same protein.

> *"In contrast to natural immunity, there are other immune responses that are stimulated by exposure to infectious agents whose magnitude and defensive capacity increase with subsequent exposure to a particular microorganism. Because this form of immunity develops in response to infection and adapts to infection, it is called adaptive or acquired immunity." Abul K. Abbas pg. 04*

Attention Adaptive immunity and acquired immunity are distinct, separate types of immunity.

Antigens- Alpha-Memory (Aa-Bb-Dd-Ee-Ff-Hh-Jj-Mm) These are all the basic antigens. These cells are part of the acquired defense system.

> *"The components of acquired immunity include lymphocytes and their products." Abul K. Abbas pg. 6*

Lymphocytes are part of the natural system, they are the parents and maternal grandparents.

ADAPTIVE IMMUNITY: EOSINOPHILS- (ALFHA -SON)

This type of immunity occurs as a last resort, so that the organism can restore itself. They are very useful in genetics, when the new embryo is constantly bombarded by enemies, especially when it comes to Alpha-Delta, and also in adulthood, when the organism is totally debilitated (this is the case with Lupo for example), then this system is activated, and all the Mater cells that are considered good or Q/B come to the aid of the individual. This group includes the Eosinophils, which are all from the Q/B group.

Eosinophils- Alfha- Son (Aa-Bb-Dd-Ff-Hh-Jj-Mm-Oo-Qq-Ss) They are the complete strand of all Q/B ending in the Mater Ss cell. Each group has its own ribbon, just as the Q/B group also has its own ribbon. Eosinophils are therefore all the good children of the Q/B group and they are constantly shat on because every eosinophil is an Alpha-Delta, so they have a high IQ and are sought after because they have a good memory, which is the main reason why they have a good memory.

be capped.

> *"all humoral and cellular immune responses to foreign antigens have certain fundamental properties that reflect the properties of the lymphocytes that mediate these responses. " Abul K. Abbas pg. 09*

There are no humoral responses; there are only three types of immune response: natural, acquired and adaptive. Secondly, antigens are part of the maternal defense cells, which you will learn more about later.

Thirdly, leukocytes are exclusively part of natural immunity.

MATER CELLS THAT ARE PART OF THE BASIC Q/B GROUP

Leukocytes
monocytes
T lymphocytes
B lymphocytes
Eosinophils
Basophiles
Enzymes
Antigens
antibodies

There are other elements in the immune system and with specific fungi

In the first group, we'll have the acid base, those self-destructive elements, and the reader will get to know who these acids are looking to destroy, a little further on.

This way, we'll find two acids trying to devour good cells.

> *"Immunology is the study of immunity in its broadest sense, that is, of the cellular and molecular events that occur after the body encounters microorganisms and other foreign macromolecules." Abul K. Andrew H. Lichtman. pg. 3*

CONCEPTUAL AND STRUCTURAL MAPPING OF THE FUNCTIONAL AND SCULPTURAL MOLD OF THE ELEMENTS THAT MAKE UP THE IMMUNE SYSTEM:

Mater Q/B Base Cells

The basic Q/B group is the favorite hunting ground of nitrous acids (macrophages and antibodies), most of which need to defend themselves against these aggressors all the time. Now the reader will understand the function of each of these elements and realize how different their function is in the body, as reported by the authors.

Leukocytes-(Aa-Bb-Cc) Who are leukocytes? They are the basic maternal grandparents and are responsible for any emergency event in the blood, blood clots, infections.

lysosine- are the pure Q/B base grands (Aa-Bb-Dd-Ff)

Polysaccharides - This is the complete strand of all the base Q/B avos (Aa- Bb-Dd-Ff-Hh-Jj-Mm-Oo-Qq-S).

Natural Killer Lymphocytes - are Q/B base avos (Aa-Bb-Dd)

Basophiles- (Aa-Bb-Dd-Ff-Hh), are sought after by acid elements because they are high IQ Alpha-Delta

T-lymphocytes (AaBb-Dd-Ff-Hh-Jj) And all Q/B tape

Neutrophils (AaBb-Dd) are the maternal grandparents

Digestive Enzymes- (Aa-Bb-Cc) are the same group of NK lymphocytes

Gayton says of neutrophils on p. 449

> *"It is mainly tissue neutrophils and macrophages that attack and destroy bacteria, viruses and other invading agents. Neutrophils are mature cells that can attack and destroy, even in circulating blood."*

About neutrophils we can say that it is the lymphocyte-like ribbon, very important of the Immune system because it is complete, so neutrophils fight incessantly to protect the cell nuclei against Reverse invaders of the Macrophage type and antibodies. Neutrophils help by gathering larger forces to protect the Q/B group.

The neutrophils are all your basic mothers, and they are there to protect rather than attack.

Eosinophils- (Aa-Bb-dd-ff-Hh-Jj-Mm-Oo-Qq-Ss) are all grandparents, and are targeted by macrophages because they all have good children.

Monocytes- (Aa- Bb-Dd-Ff) The author Gayton says once again about monocytes:

> *"Conversely, tissue macrophages begin life as monocytes in the blood, which are immature cells that, while still in the blood, have little ability to fight infectious agents." Apud pg 449.*

A monocyte would never be a macrophage because it has a base or ribbon completely opposite to macrophages.

Kerpffer cells- (Aa-Bb-Dd-Ff-Hh)

These cells are the ones that suffer the most in the immune system, they are frequent targets of attacks by macrophages. Their function is to protect the blood vessels from invaders, they provide constant protection to the blood vessels.

Macrophages (Aa-Cc-Ee-Gg-Ii-Ll-Nn-Pp-Rr-Tt-Vv-Zz)

Macrophages receive contact both from within the organism and from outside it, i.e. from individuals other than the body to which the macrophages belong, in order to phagocytize and destroy mainly cells with high IQ genes, or Alpha Delta cells, and other cells of the Q/B group, their main rivals.

In The Immune System, the reader will see that the work of antigens is the opposite of what current books explain; the antigen has a radar memory, sees a macrophage, and immediately alerts the other cells in the defense group, and they look for traps to phagocytize the foreign body.

Says the author:

> *"The most important function of neutrophils and macrophages is phagocytosis, which means cellular ingestion of the offending agent. Phagocytes must be selective as to the material that is phagocytosed, otherwise normal cells and structures of the body could be phagocytosed." Apud pg. 450*

Macrophages are specialists and know who they are looking to phagocytize, there is a specific recognition of their target which, as has already been explained, is Alpha-Delta.

Antibodies Aa-Cc-Ee-Gg-Ii-Ll-Nn)

They are also devourers of basic Q/B cells

NATURAL AND ACQUIRED IMMUNITY

> *"Natural immunity consists of cellular and biochemical defense mechanisms that already existed before the establishment of an infection, and which are programmed to respond rapidly to infections. These mechanisms have no response to non-infectious substances and respond in essentially the same way to successive infections."Apudpg*

In the natural immune system, we have the direct action of parents and maternal and paternal grandparents, all of whom belong to the Q/B group, so when an infectious process occurs, all the components of the immune system will immediately appear and, in addition to dealing with the infection, they will also be targeted by macrophages that try to prevent the action of the Q/B maternal cell group.

For a better understanding of this system, let's take a look at who is part of the natural immune defense system:

Alpha-Delta Lymphocytes - Maternal grandparents and parents (AaBb-Dd)

Alpha-Ceci- Lymphocytes are the paternal grandparents- (Aa-Bb-Dd-Ff-Hh-Jj)

It's important to point out that if we come from a group of Q/B parents and grandparents, it means that we were born into the Mother's love, and concomitantly we possess values such as faith, kindness, sincerity, and consequently we have more immunity.

Attention, there are beings who are naturally infectious, they have in their cellular formation elements so reverse, or even perverse that when they make contact with another being, it lowers the immunity of the other, decreases their energetic potential, the other feels totally unwell. A clear example of these people is their touch on a plant, the next day, there is a visible drying of that plant. Many people have given this testimony, and so have the authors. However, we don't choose to be infectious, and it doesn't depend on our actions, but on the cellular formation from which we were generated.

It's also important to point out that there are beings who come with total immunity, for life. They recognize that they are like this, which is why we hear people comment, "No disease can get to me." Others often joke, "I have a closed body and nothing can get to me". They are correct because they realize that they are immune, and indeed they are because they have the complete Q/B group cassette. They have such a good base of the Q/B group (made up of individuals with very high moral and ethical values) that they can be compared to the shell of a turtle - they have a specific molecular group, they are immune.

Acquired immunity is all the grandparents of the Q/B group.

Only parents and maternal grandparents from the Q/B group are capable of giving us immunity. When we take the vaccine, we forcibly prevent infection by damaging the components of the immune system that are deleted by the vaccine.

In the Reversas group we will meet:

Phosphoric acids

Alpha-Zebra macrophages (Aa-cc-Ee-Gg-Ii-Ll-Nn-Pp-Rr-Tt=Vv-Zz).

We then have the natural system formed by the group of Q/B mater cells, which are the target of macrophages that are real "jackals" that are constantly trying to reach, attack and capture the Alpha Delta or high Q/I. Kerpffer cells suffer the most in this story, as they try to prevent macrophages from acting on blood vessels, especially in the heart. Cytokines are great helpers in defending against enemy attacks.

It's important to know that, in the genetic system, everything is determined during fetal life, the assembly of the Q/B group determines, physical biotype, gifts (which are natural gifts), luck, and even the wealth or otherwise of an individual is already pre-established in the embryonic assembly. Thus, those cells that stand out more for their memory and other factors are also targeted by macrophages.

Thus, each human being influences their generation for up to a thousand years, which means that there is a lot of information in their genetic code, which ends up in the last twelve pairs of chromosomes.

In this way, the immune system, which is not even the right term to use, is more appropriately called the Perverse system, because at the same time as the Q/B cells are trying to protect the organism, they also need to protect themselves from the attacks of the "Jacar" macrophages. Attention, the Alpha-Mater cell exercises control over the entire organism.

We are therefore the result of our cellular complex, a group of tiny people acting on our entire organism plus everything that surrounds us, the people around us, the environment that surrounds us, in short, all of this is the result of our health or lack of it.

PROPERTIES OF THE IMMUNE RESPONSE

Antigen recognition

> *"Antigen is a substance or macromolecule, usually a protein, with the ability to induce a specific immune response. An antigen can be a genetically determined substance on the surface of a nucleated living cell or bacteria: or it can be something not directly related to any living cell. It is called endogenous if it is produced inside the host's cells and exogenous if it is produced outside them (fungi and bacteria)" Apub pg 246*

To talk about antigen recognition, let's first get to know who the antigen is, and especially its action in the immune system. The antigen is part of the set of basic maternal Q/B cells and is included in the good Q/B cells (Aa-Bb-Dd-Ff-Hh-Jj-Mm) which are the cells responsible for all the work of acquired immunity in the body.

> *"All immune responses are initiated by the specific recognition of antigens. This recognition leads to the activation of the lymphocytes that have recognized the antigen and culminates in the development of effector mechanisms that are intermediate to the physiological function of the response, i.e. the elimination of the antigen. Once the antigen has been eliminated, the immune response decreases and homeostasis is restored." Abul K. Abbas pg. 12)*

Now, an antigen is a protein with the ability to produce a specific immune response. Yes, they are responsible for clearing bacteria of viruses, of everything that is antibody, but they are a constant target for enemy attacks, as has already been explained. Antigens are the ultimate maternal sister cells. The lymphocytes recognize the antigens because they are on the same ribbon and tell them when they can be eliminated.

> *"every individual has numerous clone-derived lymphocytes, and each clone has formed from a single precursor and is capable of recognizing and responding to a distinct antigenic determinant; when the antigen enters the body, it selects a specific pre-existing clone and activates it. Foreign antigen interacts with pre-existing clones of lymphocytes specific for the antigen in the specialized lymphoid tissues in which immune responses are initiated." Abul K. Abbas pg. 13*

The clones to which the author refers are all the strands of mater cells which always start with Aa-Bb- and the lymphocytes are exactly the beginning of all the strands, i.e. Aa-Bb-Dd, but it could be; Aa- Bb- Cc, which would be the acids. So it is clear that if the antigen interacts with clones, they are not harmful to the organism.

LYMPHOCYTE ACTIVATION

> *"Lymphocytes are the only cells in the body capable of specifically recognizing and distinguishing various antigenic determinants and are therefore responsible for two defining characteristics of the acquired immune response, specificity and memory. Several lines of research have established the role of lymphocytes as the intermediate cells of acquired immunity." Abul K. Abbas pg. 18*

Lymphocytes are not part of the acquired response, and it is clear that both work together; lymphocytes are (Aa-Bb-Dd), they command the entire immune system, and consequently command antigens for some specific action, because antigens are "the cleaners" responsible for collecting all the garbage in the immune system.

> *"The function of inactive lymphocytes is to recognize antigens and initiate the acquired immune response. If it has no contact with any antigen, the cell dies through a process of apoptosis." "The nature of the self-antigens involved in lymphocyte survival is unknown." Abul K. Abbas pg.21*

This excerpt clearly shows what has been said about the action of antigens and lymphocytes. Lymphocytes are in charge, they supervise, antigens work hard to clean the organism, because of their highly trained memory, they identify where there is dirt in the organism, but they are a constant target for macrophages and antibodies. For this reason, the author says that its nature is unknown, i.e. how can antigens be a major aggressor in the body and at the same time not be?

Lymphocyte activation

> *"In the acquired immune response, inactive lymphocytes are activated by antigens and other stimuli to differentiate into effector and memory cells'Abul K. Abbas pg.23*

The antigens provide protection as memory cells, since memory cells are constant targets for enzymes and macrophages.

> *"It presents small specific regions, called epitopes responsible for the immune response or antigenic determinants that actually make contact with the antibody or other cell responsible for the immune response." Boris Osorio and Maria Regina Pg.246*

The effector phase of the immune response *"During the effector phase of the immune response, lymphocytes that have been specifically activated by antigens perform the effector functions that lead to their elimination. Antibodies and T lymphocytes eliminate extracellular and intracellular microorganisms respectively." Abul K. Abbas pg. 14*

T-lymphocytes control the elimination of microorganisms, but pay attention to the fact that antibodies are alpha-radars, they sense when there is an invasion of the organism.

MAIN CHARACTERISTICS OF THE IMMUNE RESPONSE - "IMMUNITY BLOCK"

Specificity

> *"Immune responses are specific for each antigen and even for different portions of a complex protein, a polysaccharide, or any other macromolecule. This marked specificity occurs because lymphocytes express membrane receptors on their surface that are able to distinguish discrete differences in structure between distinct antigens. " Apub Pg. 246*
>
> *"Responses to subsequent exposures to the same antigen, called secondary immune responses, generally occur more quickly, are of greater intensity and are often qualitatively different from the first response, or primary immune response to the antigen."*
>
> *"These memory cells have special characteristics that make them more efficient at eliminating the antigen than inactive lymphocytes, which have not yet been exposed to the antigen."Apub pg.246*

Antibodies

> *"Antibodies are serum proteins, of the gamma globulin type called immunoglobulins, which have paratopes or combinatorial sites (binding site of an antibody to the antigen) Antigen-antibody reactions mostly depend on mutually adjustable and specific sites, in a "lock and key" system" (Borges Osorio and Maria Regina p.247)*

Antibodies are our radars in the body, they sense when there is an invasion in the body and work together to notify the antigens, which have an excellent memory and the ability to perceive what type of bacteria is invading our body, and so they communicate via their receptors with the B or T lymphocytes, depending on the bacteria, and send a response so that they can clean up the invader. Antigens are a kind of coroner in the body, their function is to recognize a foreign body.

> *"From these studies came the more general term antibodies, to designate the plasma proteins that mediate humoral immunity. The substances that bind to antibodies and generate their production were called antigens." Abul pg.9*

There is no such thing as Humoral Immunity, the reader can see what has been written about types of immunity in this chapter, and also, antigens are constant targets for macrophages to destroy, because they provide great protection in the immune system, scouring where there are harmful organisms. Antigens are a frequent target of attack because they are recognized immediately as part of the genic group, Alpha-Delta, they have extraordinary memories and are able to detect and inform the type of invading microorganism, which is why they are the main cargo of macrophages.

Paying attention to the immune system, we can have from Aa to SS without them being reversible to the organism, but we can also have from Ee- Reversible harmful to the organism. All this depends exclusively on who makes up the strands, i.e. the molecules of each individual, which can be Reverse or Q/B. If they are Reverse, they already act as destroyers or destroy genes that are harmful to the organism, so they act in blocks.

An example of this is children who, at an early age, suffer from respiratory diseases, where no treatment is successful, or in the cardiac area, are born with serious illnesses, and it is the reverse cellular composition that promotes all this. Also, the mother can receive commands from the outside at any time during pregnancy, which leads to errors in the tapes and various deformities or illnesses.

Phagocytic cells

> *"The first cell type that enters the peripheral blood after leaving the bone marrow is already fully differentiated and is called a monocyte." "Once established in the tissues, these cells mature and become macrophages. Macrophages can exhibit different morphological forms after being activated by external stimuli, such as microorganisms." Abul Pg. 246*

Macrophages are present in all organs and in connective tissue and are given special names to designate specific locations, for example in the CNS they are called microglia, on the surface of the endothelium of the hepatic sinusoids they are called Kupffer cells; (Mind you, Kupffer cells are by no means macrophages; they protect the blood vessels, which is why they are constantly attacked), in the airways they are called alveolar macrophages and multinucleated phagocytic cells in the bones are called osteoclasts.

> *"mononuclear phagocytic cells play the role of APCs in acquired immune responses mediated by T cells." (Bores Osorio and Maria Regina P.246)*

> *"Mononuclear phagocytic cells are also important effector cells in both natural and acquired immunity." (Bores Osorio and Maria Regina P.246)*

Says the author:

> *"Thus, the components of the immune system, when a proper or not proper element is presented in a context of infection, this balance is broken and the immune response occurs." (Bores Osorio and Maria Regina P.246)*

It's difficult to talk about balance in the immune system, there are constant battles, there is an incessant search for the enemy, which is Alpha Delta.

This is not the case, as the author says: "when there is a proper or improper element". In reality, the element presented is always improper. And again: "this balance is broken and the immune response occurs". Abul K. Abbas Andrew H. Lichtman P.246

It's not a question of balance, with an immune response, it's actually a fight between some elements and others.

Acquired immune tolerance, says the author:

> *"It is the acceptance by the organism, during prenatal development or in newborns, of genetically different cells of the organism." (Boris Osorio and Maria Regina 246)*

> *"However, even non-infectious foreign substances can trigger an immunological response" Abul K. Abbas, Andrew H. Lichtman pg. 3*

Now, it's not true that any substance can trigger an immune response, that's the specific job of genes, lymphocytes and eosinophils, it depends on the need, but it's exclusively these three that participate in the immune system, in addition to macrophages that have a specific counter function in this system.

In reality, it's not a question of the organism accepting cells, but of cells with bad genes invading and taking over cells with good genes. It's not a question of immunological incompetence, as the author states, this acceptance is due to the immunological incompetence suffered by the mother cells because of the macrophage attacks.

> *"The components of acquired immunity include lymphocytes and their products. Foreign substances that induce specific immune responses or are the target of such responses are called antigens." By convention, the terms immune response and immune system refer to acquired immunity, unless otherwise specified". Abdul K. Abbas pg. 6*

Acquired immunity is carried out by antigens, which are a set of all the basic Q/B cells, the lymphocytes, and belongs to the Natural Immunity group.

It's not true that immune response and immune system refer to acquired immunity, both are distinct, specific, and acquired response is the function of antigens, while natural response is lymphocytes.

> *"T lymphocytes play central roles in all adaptive immune responses against protein antigens. In cellular immunity, CD4+ T cells activate macrophages to destroy phagocytosed microorganisms, CD4+ T helper lymphocytes destroy cells infected by intracellular microorganisms. In humoral immunity, CD4+ T helper lymphocytes interact with B lymphocytes and stimulate the proliferation and differentiation of these B lymphocytes. Both the induction phase and the effector phase of T-lymphocyte responses are triggered by the specific recognition of an antigen." Abbas, Abul K pg.83*

Mapping these two groups makes it easy to understand what is shown: **B-lymphocytes** (AaBb-Dd). T-lymphocytes (Aa-Bb-Dd-Ff-Hh-Jj) are actually the Q/B group.

Whereas **antigens are**: (Aa-Bb-Dd-Ff-Hh-Jj-Mm). They are the QB grandparents and they are sought after and captured because they are important genes. They are Alpha, Memory, because if you look at their strand, it is almost complete, so they have much more memory, and they are used as radars because they communicate with any of the strands in the Q/B group, You see, the only letter left out is the SS, or rather the last letter of the Q/B group, from this point onwards all the cells are reversed, and from this point onwards it becomes dangerous to fertilize the baby, because the rest of the cells are bad and can harm the fetus and cause many deformities. It is therefore the rest of this ribbon that produces these deformities such as Daw's Syndrome and many others.

As a result, immune responses mediated by T lymphocytes are induced only by protein antigens (the source of foreign peptides).

> *Although T lymphocytes are restricted to their own MHC, they recognize foreign MHC molecules present in tissue grafts and reject such grafts. " Abbas, Abul K pg. 85*

Note how the author refers to antigens, the source of foreign peptides, in fact they belong to an already established group of Alpha Delta that are geniuses, which is why they are sought after for capture.

Binding of antigens by antibodies

"An antigen is any substance that can be specifically bound by an antibody or by a T-cell antigen receptor."

CHAPTER IV

LUNGS: SURFACE TENSION AND JOINT ACTION OF THE CELLS IN GAS EXCHANGE

In order to understand the mechanics of lung ventilation, we need to look at the exact function of lung respiration; to begin with, we need to know that there is a very strong air pressure outside our body and that the entire process of respiration is carried out by the Mater contractile cells which are the maternal grandparents and the parents are: (Aa -b- d-f -h-j), they always walk in pairs and as a team and are responsible for the work of respiration.

> *"Principle of surface tension: the surface of the water is also trying to contract. This results in an attempt to force air out of the alveolus through the bronchus and, in doing so, induces the alveolus to collapse. The overall effect is to cause elastic contractile forcing of the whole lung which is referred to" (Guyton and Hall pg. 492).*

The surface of the water, and the force generated between the contractile cells, which are all the birds brought together in this process.

> *"Surfactant is an active agent of the water surface, which means that it greatly reduces the surface tension of the water. It is secreted by special surfactant-secreting epithelial cells called type II alveolar epithelial cells. " Guyton & Hall (Treatise on Medical Physiotherapy pg 492)*

On the process of diffusion, or "alveolar collapse", the author says:

> *"The speed of diffusion of gas molecules inside the airways is so fast, and the distances to be covered so short, that differences in concentration inside the acini are virtually abolished within a second. However, as the gas velocity drops rapidly in the region of the terminal*

bronchioles, inhaled dust often settles there."

"Pressure is caused by multiple impacts of moving molecules against a surface. Therefore, the pressure of the gas on the surfaces of the airways and alveoli is proportional to the sum of the impact forces of all the molecules of that gas that hit the surface at a given instant." (Guyton and Hall pg. 509)

The surface tension established inside the alveoli, or gas exchange, is an easy process to understand when you know who is behind it. Gas exchange does not proceed as the authors claim, but is in fact the joint work of all the mater cells, in gas exchange, or in the alveolar terminals, the only place where all twelve pairs of cells are working together.

And so, when these cells meet, it's chaos just like in the Purkinje cube, in other words, everything has to happen very quickly, like in a subway terminal, only many times faster, so as not to collapse the organism, since blood and oxygen have to be carried to the cells throughout the organism and so a cause is generated in these places, with the meeting between the two blocks of mater cells; all the grandparents in the capillaries and all the grandparents in the alveoli. The parents and grandparents or Aa, Bb, Cc, Dd, Ee and Ff are involved in the process of carrying the blood, and this works similar to a subway car in its speed carrying passengers, and thus picking up all the dirt in the body, a process carried out similar to that of a street sweeper. The Mater cells, Aa, b,c,d e, f or the grandmothers, are responsible for carrying oxygen to the alveolar terminals in order to carry oxygen to the cells throughout the body.

In this terminal, there is a very fast process between these cells, where the "metro sangue" quickly throws the Co2 collected by the "garis" and even faster picks up the O2 from the grandmothers, who are terrified by the gas received and the agitation of the high-speed exchange. The exchange is carried out at such a high speed that there appears to be dust, as the author claims, and he also says that the speed of the gas drops, when this is not true.

In the chordae tendineae, in the trabeculae carnea, in the musculus pectineae, which are actually cubes, unlike the nodes which are tubes, we have these cubes which will house the mater cells always in a division similar to what has already been described. In the chordae tendineae, the quartet is in the tricuspid, and looks like three cusps, but Aa and B, are together in one block, followed by C and D., so they are together in this process, they are the parents and grandparents together, then come the Reversals; Ee and Ff are in the bicuspid, in the ventricles, the mater quartet is in the right ventricle while the garis cells are in the left ventricle doing the heaviest work which is to send oxygenated blood to the whole body, in the lungs, the mater cells are in the right lobe or right tubes, which are three tubes, in the left tubes, are the peoes, which are in charge of receiving and sending oxygen to the capillaries.

Thus, the two trios always work in opposition, following the cardiac cycle (systole and diastole) which ends in pulmonary oxygenation or hematosis, between these two vital organs; heart and lung, thus setting up a closed circle between them.

In the lungs, the inhalation and exhalation continue the cardiac cycle, the behavior of the maternal cells is the same as already mentioned, in the three lobes or pulmonary cubes, where only the mothers and maternal grandmothers work together and are distributed as follows

1st pulmonary cube; QB mater cells Aa, Bb, second pulmonary cube, Cc, Dd and in the third cube Ee and Ff. On the left side, which contains two "lobes" or cubes, just like in the heart, they are distributed as follows: In the first cube, Aa, Bb, Cc, Dd, in the second tube Ee- Ff.

Note: Nodal tissue is a property of constant stimulation where contractile cells function. Purkinje or all the grandparents together, Mater Aa-Bb -Dd- Cc- f cells, carry out the systole and filling process in the heart and are responsible for the formation of twins.

In the respiratory system, the effects of LS on chronic obstructive pulmonary disease (COPD) are a reminder of the danger posed by the action of waste on the functioning of the body as a whole, which has been responsible for a very high percentage of illnesses that lead to death, not in the short term, but in conditions that are often irreversible, especially when it comes to respiratory diseases, since the lungs are one of the main organs responsible for purifying the body and it becomes difficult to remove the LS deposited in the pulmonary alveoli.

> *"Respiratory failure is currently one of the most serious problems in intensive care units around the world. The mortality rate ranges from 21% to 75%, depending on the region". (MACHADO, 2008, p. 171).*

Respiratory failure is characterized by the inability to maintain adequate gas exchange with the ambient air, either due to incorrect supply of oxygen to the tissues or inadequate elimination of carbon dioxide by the lungs, in both cases, we see the action of the LS.

Airway dysfunction can occur due to internal obstruction, of which L S is the champion in terms of obstruction of the internal walls of the airways. Any author dealing with this subject claims oxygenation failure with hypoxemia mechanisms including low oxygen tension in the inspired air, diffusion disturbance and the ventilation-perfusion ratio.

In reality, there are people who receive more or less of this load of garbage, and if there is more, it will be difficult for oxygen to enter the alveoli, which will be impeded by the LS, and consequently there will be a disturbance in the diffusion of oxygen. First of all, it's important to know about the function of the lungs in order to understand how LS acts in this process, i.e. in the distribution of oxygen to the gas exchange surface, where carbon dioxide or LS is discharged into the atmosphere. Thus, the air is carried by a directed flow into the alveoli and distributed to the gas exchange surface, where diffusion carries out the exchange process. Transport through the airways depends on the permeability of the tubes, the compliance of the lungs and the strength of the respiratory muscles, as well as the deposit of LS in the alveoli and the bloodstream, where LS is also carried. In chronic bronchitis, obstruction occurs due to thickening of the bronchial mucosa and the presence of secretion, while in emphysema it is different: the elastic structure that maintains the radial trachea over the airways is weakened. In both cases we see the action of LS; it destroys the walls, whether alveolar or pulmonary, and also acts on the formation of the mucosa.

Chronic and acute bronchitis are CLINICAL SYNDROMES characterized by a chronic or acute cough with mucous or mucopurulent sputum lasting for months and a reduction in forced expiratory volume.

This study also shows the action of LS in COPD, so the movement of molecules will be observed as fundamental proof of the movement of LS and its action in the body. This research is contrary to what the authors write about the movement of molecules under gas pressure. According to Hall:

> *"Gases dissolved in water or body tissues also exert pressure because the dissolved gas molecules move randomly and have kinetic energy" (HALL, 2011, p. 509).*

The molecules don't move randomly, this process involves the five units of mater cells, or twelve pairs of cells that have kinetic energy and face each other, and they receive pressure from each other, where the Alpha, Beta, Ceci and Delta cells are fighting against the Reversas performing their carrier function. the molecules "go crazy" trying to survive, so it is not true what the author justifies, they are hit as in a bombing, defending themselves as much as they can.

"Pressure is caused by multiple impacts of moving molecules against a surface" (HALL, 2011, p. 509). The multiple impacts of the molecules are, as mentioned above, the struggle between the contractile cells, where some end up deteriorating.

Factors that determine the partial pressure of gas dissolved in liquid.

"Some types of molecules, especially carbon dioxide molecules, are physically or chemically attracted to water molecules, while others are repelled."

According to Hall:

On the other hand, molecules of the same gas that are already dissolved in the blood move randomly in the blood liquid, and some of these molecules move and escape back into the alveoli. The speed with which they escape is directly proportional to their partial pressure in the blood (HALL, 2011, p. 510).

The author himself confirms what was explained earlier: "some of these moving molecules escape back into the alveoli" (HALL, 2011, p. 510). So it is not true that the speed with which they escape is directly proportional to the pressure faced between the contractile cells.

The author says about water and steam pressure:

"This results from the fact that water molecules, as well as those of dissolved gases, are continuously escaping from the surface of the water into the gaseous phase. The partial pressure exerted by the water molecules to escape from the surface is called the water vapor pressure." Apub Hall pg 510

The surface is actually the pressure of the water vapor. The partial pressure is the water molecules trying to escape from the gas molecules, so it would be fairer to say that it is the pressure between the contractile cells themselves.

"It is clear that when the gas pressure is higher in one area than in the other, there will be effective diffusion from the high-pressure area to the low-pressure area; however, some molecules will agitate randomly from the low-pressure area to the high-pressure area. (Guyton&Hall, 2011, p. 510)"

Regarding the composition of alveolar air and atmospheric air, the author makes a comparison showing that alveolar air does not have the same concentrations as atmospheric air and gives 4 reasons for this: partial substitution by atmospheric air, oxygen absorbed by the pulmonary blood, carbon dioxide going from the lungs to the alveoli.

"The faster oxygen is absorbed, the lower its concentration in the alveoli; the faster oxygen is breathed into the alveoli from the atmosphere, the higher its concentration." (HALL, 2011, p. 512).

"Therefore, the concentrations and partial pressures of both oxygen and carbon dioxide in the alveoli are determined by the intensity of absorption or excretion of the two gases and the value of alveolar ventilation" (HALL, 2011, p. 513).

CHAPTER V

General principles of the unified nervous and muscular system

This book brings together many new concepts in neurology, showing that this system is very important in maintaining the harmonious functioning of the skeleton, since the contractile mater cells are very active here, always acting with great precision and coherence. The other systems are somewhat intertwined with this one, especially the muscular system, which is directly linked to the nervous system.

Energetic Circulatory Sensory System - Aa-Bb (Alpha-Beta)
Sensory control system of the MCCs (Mater Contractile Cells) Aa- Bb-Dd
Circulatory System (blood, lymphatic, hormonal, respiratory) Aa-Bb- Dd-Ff-Hh-Jj
Articular Skeletal System Aa-Bb-Cc-Dd-Ee-Ff
Immune system and genetics unified Aa-Bb-Dd-Ff-Hh-Jj-Mm-Oo-Qq-Ss- Uu-Xx
Unified nervous and muscular system Aa-Bb-Cc-Dd-Ee-Ff-Gg-Ii
The senses are:
Afferent Sensory Senses Aa- Bb (Alpha and Beta)
Skin senses (touch, pressure, vibration, cold, heat, pain, itching) Aa-Bb-Dd-Ff
Sense of smell Aa- Bb- Cc
Sense of hearing Aa-Bb-Dd
Taste Aa-Bb-Dd
Optical direction- Aa-Bb-Cc

The classification of Nerves is:

Seven ribbons in pairs

1ª tape- Oculomotor nerve- Aa-Bb (Alpha and Delta)
2ª tape- Olfactory and optic nerves Aa-Bb-Cc
3rd ribbon- Torclear nerve Aa- Bb-Cc-Ee

4th tape - Nerves - trigeminal, facial, vestibular - Aa-Bb-Dd
5th ribbon- Nerves- Abducent,Accessory- Aa-Bb-Dd-Ff
6th ribbon- Nerves- accessory, vagus- Aa-Bb-Cc-Ee-Gg-Ii
7th Ribbon- Hypoglossal nerve- Aa-Bb-Dd-Ff-Hh

The Nervous System is the third most important system in the body, since it is responsible for measuring all the information that enters and leaves the body in order to process consciousness, cognition, memory, intelligence, ethics and behavior, with control of all movement, action and reaction throughout the body, through the command of the MCCs.

> *"The most important role of the nervous system is to control the various activities of the body. This function is performed by controlling the contraction of the appropriate skeletal muscles throughout the body, the contraction of the musculature"*

> *"The nervous system is unique in the vast complexity of the cognitive processes and control actions it can perform. Every minute it receives literally millions of bits of information from different organs and sensory nerves and then integrates them to determine the responses to be executed by the body." Hall and John, pg. 571 treatise of medical physiology Rio de janeiro 2011.*

In Neurology, until now we had known about three neurons acting in the entire nervous system, but what we have is a joint work carried out by three pairs of Mater cells that do all the work in the entire central nervous system.

Angelo Machado says:

> *"We have seen how the three fundamental neurons already present in anetodes appeared during phylogenesis: the afferent neuron, the efferent neuron and the association neuron. Angelo Machado pg. 04*

Afferent neuron

> *"It arose in phylogenesis with the function of providing the central nervous system with information about changes in the external environment...The receptors, capable of transforming the various types of physical or chemical stimuli into nerve impulses, which are conducted to the central nervous system by the sensory neuron. " (Angelo Machado pg. 04 - 05)*

The afferent neurons are made up of three pairs of mater cells, which are the parents and two grandparents QB Aa-Bb-Dd they do not receive and carry information, their function is to form axes, they are a kind of lamp that lights up, they illuminate the idea.

Efferent Neuron - However, the efferent neurons that innervate smooth muscles, cardiac muscles or glands have their bodies outside the central nervous system, in structures that are the visceral ganglia.

The efferent neurons are the paternal grandparents and are responsible for the conduction of the augurs.

Sao Aa-Bb-Cc-Ee

Association neuron

> *"The body of the association neuron always remains within the central nervous system and its number has increased greatly during evolution." (Angelo Machado pg. 04 - 05)*

There is no such thing as an association neuron, they are a single set of five pairs of mater cells responsible for all the work in neurology.

I Neuron: formed by the maternal grandparents: Aa- Bb-Dd (Alpha Beta Delta)
II Neurons are formed by the paternal grandparents: Aa-Bb-Cc-Ee (Alpha, Beta Ceci, Reverse E)
Neurons are all grandparents together: Aa-Bb-Cc-Dd-Ee-Ff

Lower neuron: The paternal grandparents Aa Cc Ee (Alpha Ceci E Reversa)
Upper Neuron: All maternal grandparents Aa-Bb-Dd-Ff (Alpha Beta, Delta, Hexa Mater)
Afferent pathway: All paternal grandparents Aa-Bb-Dd (Alpha, Beta and Delta)

Efferent Pathway: The maternal grandparents Aa-Bb-Dd- (Alpha, Beta, Delta,)

Through the major afferent pathways, which are carried out by the formation of all the basic QB avos.

While in the efferent pathway are the parents and maternal grandparents Aa-Bb-Dd- we can also observe the movement of LS in the body and thus find some flaws, due to the authors' lack of knowledge about this substance that has so degraded and mutilated human beings. The major afferent pathways are considered to be the ones that carry impulses coming from the receptors to the super-food nerve centers.

We won't be looking at the routes in this study, as this wouldn't be the aim of the research, but rather clarifying the entry of the LS into this system.

Starting with its movement in the Bulb where what is called the **Bulbar Olive**, which are **bulbar calluses**, a resistance offered by six maternal and paternal grandparents: Aa-Bb-Cc-Dd-Ee-Ff to prevent the passage of this garbage. The midbrain is also attacked by the LS, which causes difficulties in the synapses.

AFFERENT AND EFFERENT PATHWAYS IN THE NEW FUNCTIONAL MOLD

The first neuron in the periphery, formed by a sensitive ganglion, is made up of the maternal Aa-Bb-Dd grandparents where the peripheral extension joins the receptor and the central extension goes to the CNS via the dorsal roots of either the spinal or cranial nerve. This is where synapses occur, via neurons, which are nothing more than the continuation of the mother cells.

The lower motor neuron is formed by the parents Alfha and the paternal grandparents Aa- Cc-Ee , which is responsible for distributing the information received directly to the muscles, while the upper neurons are formed by the mater cells, Alfha, Beta, Delta- Aa-Bb-Dd

Neuron II is located in the posterior column of the spinal cord or in the nuclei of the cranial nerves of the brainstem and is formed by the paternal grandparents: Aa- Cc-Ee (Alfha, Ceci, E Reversa,) form axons and enter the formation of a tract or leminiscus.

Attention - There is no third neuron, it is the work of the same set of Mater cells.

An axon that passes through the inner capsule, the corona radiata, making a synapse in the cerebral cortex. In this region, all the information about anger, rage and pain that reaches this region is processed.

To summarize, we can say that this region is the second great garbage dump of the body, where the first takes place in the bulb, a place called bulbar olives, but which are actually bulbar calluses.

From there we found the key to the various illnesses processed in the brain causing degeneration in the cellular body, and which current science has been unable to explain and give concrete answers to certain illnesses such as: Alzheimer's, multiple sclerosis, Parkinson's and epilepsy, this being a response of the cardiac system, together with the drop in sodium and potassium that ends up causing a heating of the mind, and the triggering of convulsions. as explained before.

Therefore, the conscious proprioception pathway that is formed by the phosphoric acid; Aa-Cc-Ee.

> *"Neuron III is located in the ventral posterolateral nucleus of the thalamus, originating axons that constitute thalamic radiations that reach the somesthetic area passing through the internal capsule and radiated crown. (...) The impulses that follow this route become conscious exclusively at the cortical level". (MACHADO, 2006, p. 288)*

CHAPTER VI

THE LARGEST SYSTEM; CENTRAL ENERGETIC SENSORY SYSTEM, MADE UP OF:

Purkinje cells AaBbDd
Deep nuclear cells AaBb
Granule cells Aa Bb Dd Ff
Alpha (Aa) Beta (Bb) Delta (Dd) Hexa Mater (Ff)

1-Purkinje distributed energy chain

No scientific study has dealt with this system, yet it is the most important system in the whole organism, because it is the system on which the vitality of cells, conductivity and final definitions of any event depend, especially in genetics. We're talking about the Purkinje cells, which are responsible for the entire energetic sensory system in our organism. They define the entire conduction of the embryo through the process of conductivity. In reality, purkinje is the deep nuclear cell.

> *"The output of the Functional Unit comes from a deep nuclear cell. This cell is continuously under excitatory and inhibitory influences. Excitatory influences originate from direct connections with afferent fibers that enter the cerebellum from the central nervous system or from the periphery. The inhibitory influence originates entirely from the Purkinje cell in the cerebellar cortex." (Page 701 Guyton and Hall, Treatise on Medical Physiology 2006 Rio de Janeiro)*

The fibers in vines, as the author explains, are part of the energetic sensory system, or rather the purkinje cells. They appear in the lower olives of the bulb, they are energy channels, which will be circulating throughout the body, they are just confused by the authors who change their denomination in various segments of the organism. What the authors call climbing cells, are in fact the purkinje command, in the form of a ray; they come out in the form of deep nuclear cells, they appear as purkinje, climbing cells, granule cells, but they are in fact the Alpha, Beta and Delta cells at work.

> *"After sending branches to several deep nuclear cells, the climbing fiber continues its journey to the outer layers of the cerebellar cotex, where it makes around 300 synapses with the cell body and dendrites of each Purkinje cell. These climbing fibers are distinguished by the fact that a single nerve will always cause a single, characteristic and prolonged action potential in each purkinje cell, starting with a powerful cell followed by a set of weaker cells. This action potential is called a complex molecule." (Page 702 Guyton and Hall, Treatise on Medical Physiology 2006 Rio de Janeiro)*

So what we see is a chain process of the energy circle, formed by Alpha, Beta and Delta cells, which the authors call purkinje cells, climbing cells, mossy cells, deep nuclear cells.

> *"A characteristic of Purkinje cells and deep nuclear cells is that both fire continuously, the Purkinje cell firing about 50 to 100 action potentials per second, and the deep nuclear cells at higher rates." (Page 702 Guyton and Hall, Treatise on Medical Physiology 2006 Rio de Janeiro)*

> *"It should be noted that direct stimulation of deep nuclear cells by climbing and mossy fibers causes their excitation." (Page 702 Guyton and Hall, Treatise on Medical Physiology 2006 Rio de Janeiro)*

So it's a closed chain circle of just three pairs of cells.[

FINAL CONSIDERATIONS

Through this study, we present to the scientific community two new concepts, totally unprecedented, and which will greatly help in the knowledge of certain diseases that are still obscure in the medical literature; **Sitiating Garbage and Mater Contractile Cells,** very important for their action in three systems; Circulatory, Immune System and Genetics, but they are not the only ones, garbage is found in the seven systems of the organism, in the same way that Mater Contractile Cells, which are control cells, are found in all vital systems. This study explains a new paradigm on how the control of five units of cells that always work in antithesis and in a closed circle in pairs, as a team, in a precise and coherent way, which we call **Mater Contractile Cells**, is processed in our organism, due to the fact that these cells are specialized, receive and issue afferent and efferent commands and are in all seven vital systems of our organism, they act according to the system; in the immune system and in genetics, they are the only systems where these cells work in their entirety; 23 pairs of cells or 23 pairs of chromosomes, where in reality this study has explained countless times that there are 24 pairs of cells, where the first of them has two in one.

These cells work in ten systems: in the heart they are responsible for the cardiac cycle, in the lungs for gas exchange, in the nerves for synapses, in the muscles for contraction, in the blood for cleansing the organism, in respiration for gas exchange in genetics, they do all the work of reproduction, they form the genetic code, they give the embryo its characteristics and they are also responsible for gene duplication.

This study clearly defines both concepts, stating that they are the key and the lock to understanding or explaining countless diseases in any part of the body.
LS is responsible for a multitude of pathologies, and this study answers many questions raised in the current medical literature, from cancer, diabetes, rheumatological infections and other pathologies lodged in the human body.

Lixo Sitiante is therefore a cosmic dust that appears in the form of a gray mass in the body, like cement dust on a leaf, and so it appears in the cell acting as a very potent poison affecting the structure of the cellular system whether in the membrane, the synovial fluid, the ligaments, or even inside the cell in its various segments. It enters man through the sacral foramen up to L5, becoming invasive at this point, in the spinal cord where it accompanies the cerebrospinal fluid that runs longitudinally through it, bridging the brainstem and reaching the arachnoid granules through the superior sargital sinus and thus falling into the bloodstream, acting in a chain from there on seven systems in our organism, namely: Bone, muscle, integumentary, circulatory, immune, respiratory and genetic systems.

In Genetics, LS modifies the cell's DNA, causing mutations, errors in the various stages of transcription and translation, causing structural changes in the DNA, or simply DN. Thus, chromosomal abnormalities arise, including: Trisomy 21 (Down's Syndrome); Trisomy 18 Syndrome, Trisomy 13 Syndrome, where the authors of this event say that the underlying cause of the non-disjunction in the event is unclear, claiming that Down's is more common in the offspring of older mothers. In reality, at an older age there is a greater accumulation of LS in the body, which you will understand better as you get to know this study.

In the brain, LS, which is responsible for removing sodium from the body, causes various types of damage such as Alzhaimer's disease, dementia, Parkson's disease, multiple sclerosis, forgetfulness, slowness and the many deformities described in the medical literature.

Maternal Contractile Cells

Our whole body works in **antithesis** and in a **closed circle**, but the ones responsible for this intense work are five pairs of cells (**Mater Contractile Cells**) which are part of a larger group of command cells, the way they act in the body is still unknown to current science. Therefore, MCCs are a tiny population that acts on seven systems in our body, namely: Bone system, muscular system, integumentary system, circulatory system, immune system, respiratory system and genetics. This tiny population is always working

These cells answer questions about countless diseases, and deformities too, which will be seen in Genetics.

REFERENCES

HALL, John E. **Treatise on Medical Physiology.** 12ª ed. Rio de Janeiro: Elsevier, 2011.

MACHADO, Maria da Gloria Rodrigues. **Bases of Respiratory Physiotherapy.** 1st ed. Rio de Janeiro: Guanabara Koogan, 2008.

Borges Osorio and Maria Regina- genetica humana 2nd edition Porto Alegre: Ed artmed 2001

Fisioterapia Reumatologica/ Berenice chiarello, PatriciaDriusso, Andre Luis Maiera Radi

Barueri, Sao Paulo, Manole, 2005

Physiotherapy manuals

Kapandji, A I Joint physiology: Trunk and spine. Ed Guanabara Sao Paulo 2000 p. 74 a122

Article- Brazilian Fibromyalgia Consensus- 25 authors p. 57 to 65:

Brazilian Journal of Prescription and Exercise Physiology

ISSN 1981-9900 Electronic version

Article- Physical activity in improving the quality of life of fibromyalgia patients Priscilla de Miranda Carvalho p. 47 to 566

Skare, TL Rheumatology: Principles and Practices. Rio de Janeiro- Guanabara Koogan, 1999-p. 73,77

Dario Doretto- Clinical Pathophysiology of the Nervous System Fundamentals of

Semiology 2ª Edi Atheneu Rio de JaneirogO

Mouth breathing and body posture, a cause and effect relationship Andrea Verissimo Reis Costa

Rio de Janeiro 19999

Cardio-vascular physiology

Publisher: Paulo j f Tucci

p. 47 to 63

Guyton & Hall, Treatise on Medical Physiology,

12th Edition Rio de Janeiro 20011

Elsevier 2011

Abulk K Abbas Andrew H. Lichtman- Cellular and Molecular Immunology 5th Edition Rio de Janeiro 2005

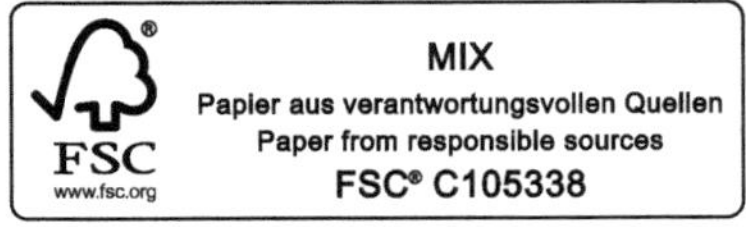

Printed by Books on Demand GmbH, Norderstedt / Germany